Paleo Meal Prep

Weekly Meal Plans and Recipes to
Eat Healthy at Work, Home, or On the Go

Paleo Meal Prep

by Kenzie Swanhart

Photography by Laura Flippen

ROCKRIDGE
PRESS

For general information on our other products and services or to obtain technical support, please contact our Customer Care Department within the United States at (866) 744-2665, or outside the United States at (510) 253-0500.

Rockridge Press publishes its books in a variety of electronic and print formats. Some content that appears in print may not be available in electronic books, and vice versa.

Interior and Cover Designer: Brieanna Hattey Felschow
Art Producer: Karen Williams
Editor: Rachelle Cihonski
Production Editor: Andrew Yackira

Photography © 2020 Laura Flippen

Author photo courtesy of © Julien Levesque

ISBN: Print 978-1-64739-617-6 | eBook 978-1-64739-385-4

R0

For my mom, thank you for teaching me
to always chase my dreams.

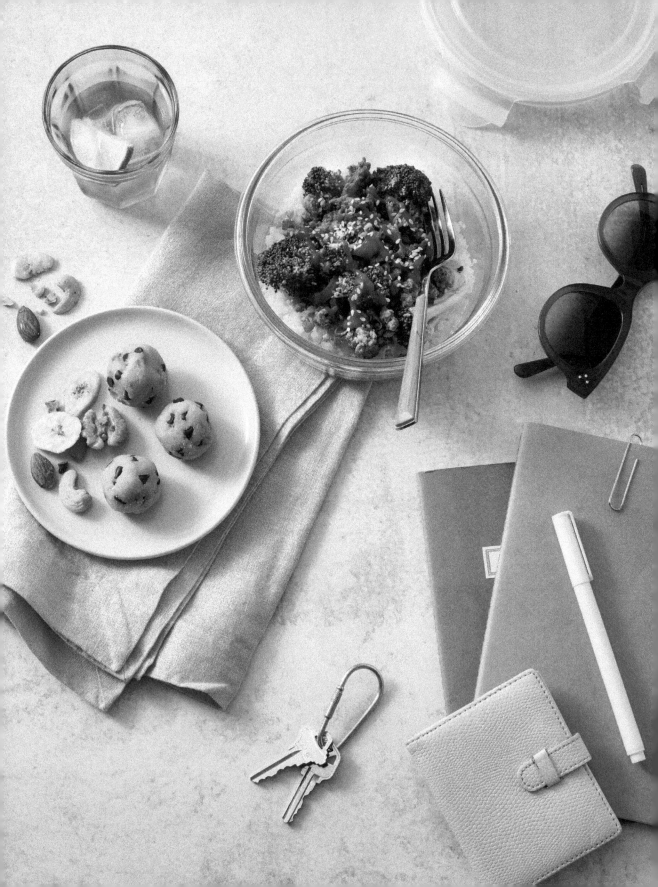

Contents

Introduction

I am lucky enough to spend my days writing and testing recipes, talking about food, and teaching others about cooking. Despite my passion for food, cooking during the week often becomes a source of stress and aggravation. After all, I am often so busy trying to get everything done, that what to eat for lunch or cook for dinner frequently falls to the bottom of the list.

Enter meal prep. You have likely seen beautifully arranged containers of pre-prepped meals flooding your social media feed. Not only is meal prep popular because the meals are pretty to look at, but they are convenient as well. There's no need to stress about what to make for dinner or to reach for the takeout menu when you have a delicious meal prepped and ready to eat in the refrigerator. By planning and prepping your meals in advance, you are guaranteed to have nutritious meals ready when you want to eat. Meal prep is the answer for those who want to eat healthy and save money—who want to know what they'll be eating each week, and to enjoy healthy meals without spending every night in the kitchen. Best of all, meal prep doesn't have to be a daunting task. Unfortunately, deciding what to prep and how to store it isn't exactly intuitive. That is why I wrote this book!

About eight years ago I adopted a Paleo lifestyle as a way to improve my health, feel better, and learn new things in the kitchen. I followed a strict Paleo lifestyle for about five years; however, over the past few years I had trouble sticking to it. I reintroduced non-Paleo approved foods back into my diet, I started eating out more, and ultimately, I was cooking recipes and teaching folks how to cook who did not follow a Paleo lifestyle.

Once again, I was feeling sluggish, relying on coffee to keep me going throughout the day. I felt bloated and was having digestive issues and migraines—just all around not my best. That's when I decided to jump back into the Paleo diet, but I knew I needed to find a way to make it easier to follow.

I know that eating Paleo can be a challenge. It can be time-consuming to make your own food every day with clean, fresh ingredients. That is why I started meal prepping. By taking the time to plan and cook my meals for the week in advance, I am able to stay on track despite how busy life gets.

This is the reason I decided to write this book—to help others who are attempting the switch to a Paleo lifestyle, or are just trying to eat better by meal prepping for the week. I have learned a lot and I can't wait to share my tips and tricks with you. Not only does this book provide you with all the background knowledge you need to understand exactly what eating Paleo means, but it takes the guesswork out of what to prep for the week. I have included a variety of simple, budget-friendly recipes that can be made in advance and enjoyed throughout the week, as well as meal plans that range from getting started on Paleo, to those using Paleo to fuel or maintain their lifestyle. Remember: A little prep in advance will save you a ton of time during the week and will keep you on track to meet your goals. Pretty soon, you'll be well on your way to eating Paleo, and enjoying more time outside of the kitchen.

Whether you are looking to lose weight, improve your health, or spend less time in the kitchen, meal prepping Paleo meals can help you accomplish your goals. So, what are you waiting for? Grab your apron and arrange your storage containers—it's time to meal prep!

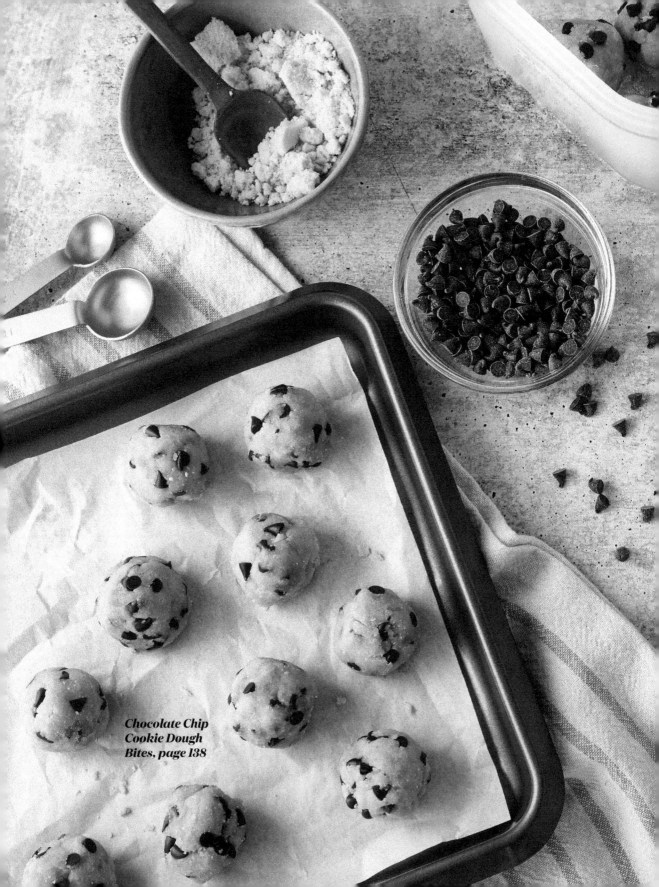

**Chocolate Chip
Cookie Dough
Bites, page 138**

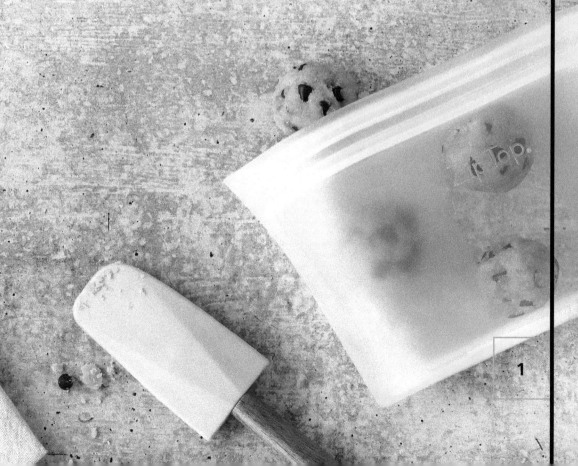

PART 1

Meal Prep Goes Paleo

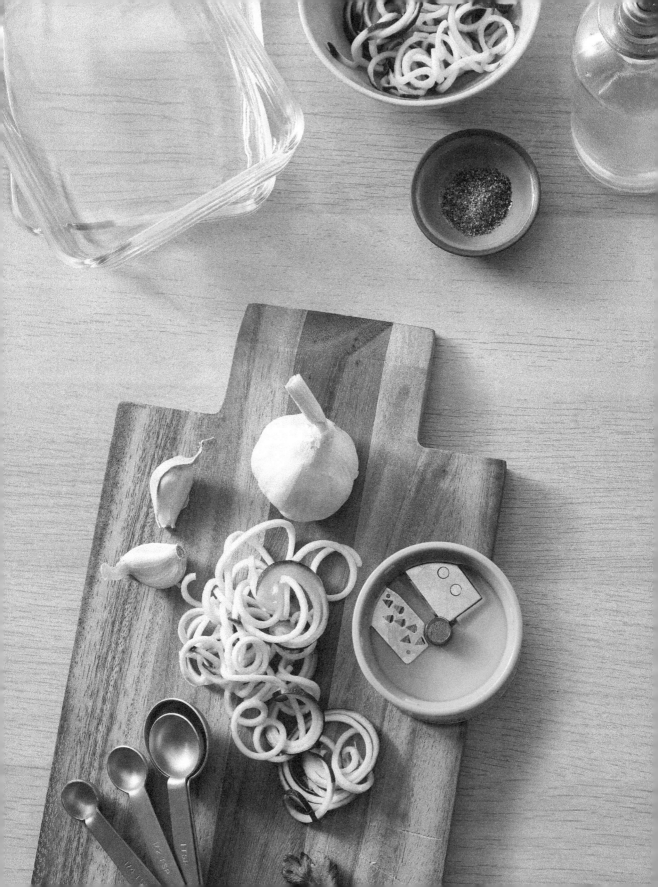

CHAPTER 1

On-the-Go Paleo

When I first started following a Paleo lifestyle, I was excited to dive right in. One of the most important things I discovered, however, is the more you know and the more prepared you are, the less intimidating this new lifestyle will be.

Enter meal prep. With some forethought and a few hours of prep, you can have a week's worth of healthy, balanced meals in the refrigerator ready to grab, reheat, and eat. Whether you are new to Paleo and looking to simplify your transition to a Paleo diet, or you are looking for new and delicious prep-able meals to add to your weekly repertoire, meal prep will take the hassle out of Paleo cooking and the guesswork out of your week. Furthermore, understanding the principles behind the Paleo diet and how to apply them to your everyday routine will help guide you toward a healthy, balanced lifestyle.

This chapter will provide a primer on how to meal prep for the Paleo diet like a pro, and includes an overview of the principles of Paleo, as well as tips and best practices for meal prep. Get ready to be a Paleo meal prep master in no time.

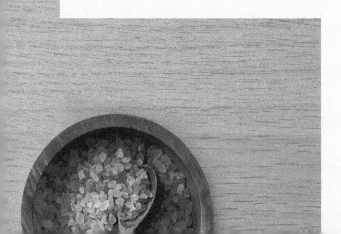

The Pros of Meal Prep

I love to cook almost as much as I love to eat, but I'm not a fan of spending hours in the kitchen during the week. I work long hours, and I want to eat well with as little effort as possible.

The power of meal prep is that it can streamline your week, reduce stress, and eliminate the hectic "what's for dinner" debate. It will also help you maintain your health and fitness goals by removing the temptation to grab something easier and non-Paleo when you're in a hurry.

This book will take the fear out of meal prepping, saving you time and energy in the process. Below are five of the major benefits of meal prep.

1. **It saves you time.** Imagine cooking just once a week. While you might spend a few hours cooking over the weekend, you'll have more free time on your weeknight evenings. You'll dirty, wash, dry, and put away pots and pans once instead of nightly. The only nightly dishes you'll have are those used to store your pre-portioned meals. To save even more time when meal prepping: Take everything out when you get started so you can see all of the ingredients and tools you need, choose some pre-prepped ingredients so you can save on chopping time, and freeze half of the batch so you have easy to reheat-and-eat freezer meals.

2. **It saves you money.** Meal prepping and portioning your meals is one of the easiest and most effective ways to manage your food budget. The process requires you to write out a specific grocery list, which saves you from purchasing impulse items or unnecessary ingredients during your shopping trips; this also means less food waste, a win-win for you and the environment! You will also be less tempted to reach for the takeout menu or spend money going out to dinner when you have a delicious, healthy meal waiting for you in the refrigerator. When getting started, you may have some upfront expenses if you don't have ingredients like extra-virgin olive oil, spices, and other staples in your pantry. However, these ingredients will be used for many meals, saving you money over time.

3. **It makes healthy eating easier.** Folks in the health and fitness space have been doing meal prep for a long time, and for good reason. It is well known

that cooking at home means you control the ingredients in your meals. Therefore, food prepared at home is often healthier because you are using whole ingredients and consuming fewer carbohydrates, less sugar, less sodium, and less fat. It also means that it is easier to follow a specific diet or way of eating because you are actually choosing, buying, and cooking each ingredient. I like to meal prep delicious meals that are often a twist on my favorite comfort and takeout foods so that I am excited to eat the meals I have prepped. After all, you aren't going to want to eat a meal you've prepared if it isn't food you enjoy.

4. **It provides portion control.** Perhaps the most obvious benefit of meal prepping is that your meals have built-in portion control. Each meal is measured out and placed in a storage container so that you can grab and go or grab and reheat. When you don't have leftovers sitting on the stove, you are less likely to go back for seconds.

5. **It reduces stress.** You make so many decisions throughout the day that sometimes it feels like one more choice will leave you paralyzed. At the same time, my husband and I are trying to answer the question, "What's for dinner?" Planning and cooking dinner can be the most stressful time of the day, but it doesn't have to be! Plan and prep in advance, and you will already know what is for dinner each night, no last-minute decision making required.

The Paleo Diet Principles

You have probably heard the Paleo diet called a lot of things: primal, real food, clean eating, the caveman diet, and the hunter-gatherer diet, among others. Simply put, eating Paleo refers to eating the way our ancestors once did—specifically in the Paleolithic, pre-agricultural era. That means ditching the modified, processed junk foods often consumed in the modern American diet and replacing them with the whole, clean foods we were designed to eat.

The foods our ancestors ate mainly consisted of lean meats, vegetables, some fruit, a little bit of starch, and good, healthy fats. These are the foods we are genetically wired to consume, the foods that will help us maintain healthy, active lifestyles.

Paleo is not a fad diet; it is a lifestyle built on consuming the foods that were meant to fuel our bodies. Though Paleo seems like a relatively new lifestyle, it has actually been around for several decades. Food tribes are now on the rise, and Paleo rose to popularity when people started looking for a healthy, sustainable way to lose weight, improve their health, and achieve a balanced lifestyle. People have continued to eat this way because it makes them feel good, and that is why I choose to follow a Paleo lifestyle.

While all versions of the Paleo diet follow the same premise, it's important to remember that this diet is not one-size-fits-all, nor is there a single list of foods that works best for everyone. Over time, you will discover which foods are optimal for you and your goals.

Paleo Approved or Off the Table?

Understanding what you can and cannot eat on the Paleo diet is important and can be difficult in the modern era. After all, our Paleolithic ancestors did not have to navigate supermarkets filled with temptation.

Here are the basics: Eat real food, including meat, seafood, eggs, vegetables, fruits, and good fats from oils, nuts, and seeds. Eat natural, unprocessed foods with very few ingredients (or better yet, no added ingredients at all). When in doubt, read the list of ingredients. If you can't pronounce something, don't eat it. It's as simple as that.

Choosing whole fruits and vegetables may come easy given they are naturally unprocessed, but what about other foods that are less obvious? Here is a helpful list to help you navigate these foods. This list is not exhaustive, but should be used as a basic guideline.

Paleo Approved

Proteins Lean cuts of meat, especially from grass-fed animals, including beef, pork, chicken, lamb, and turkey, are a staple of the Paleo diet. When consuming fish and shellfish, wild caught is always preferred on the Paleo diet. Other Paleo-approved sources of protein include bacon, bison, duck, and venison.

Vegetables Seasonal fresh vegetables should be the foundation of most meals on the Paleo diet. Be sure to follow the Clean Fifteen and Dirty Dozen (ewg.org) when choosing which vegetables to buy organic. I also keep a few bags of frozen veggies in the freezer for emergencies. Vegetables I use frequently include asparagus, beets, broccoli, carrots, cauliflower, celery, eggplant, mushrooms, onions, parsnips, spinach, squash, sweet potatoes, and zucchini.

Fruits Fruits can be a great way to satisfy your sweet tooth and should be enjoyed in moderation. I also keep a few bags of frozen fruit and berries in the freezer year-round. I like to keep a variety of fruits on hand, including apples, avocados, bananas, berries, cucumbers, lemons, limes, mangos, pears, pineapples, tomatoes, and watermelon, among others. Dried fruit can also be enjoyed on the Paleo diet; look for options with no added sugar.

Eggs Eggs are a great source of protein and are a staple of the Paleo diet.

Healthy Fats Healthy fats are a crucial component of the Paleo diet. Beyond what you consume from protein, opt for healthy fats when cooking and baking, such as organic grass-fed butter and ghee, coconut oil, avocado oil, olive oil, lard, and tallow.

Herbs and Spices Use dried or fresh herbs and spices to add flavor to your dishes. Experiment with new flavors and consider that many herbs and spices offer health benefits and properties.

Nuts and Seeds Nuts and seeds taste great and can be used to add texture and flavor to a dish. I like to keep almonds, cashews, pecans, pumpkin seeds, and sesame seeds on hand. They can also be transformed into delicious nut butters.

Natural Sweeteners Many people following the Paleo diet avoid sweeteners, but not all sweeteners are created equal. While baking and cooking, opt for natural sweeteners like agave, pure maple syrup, molasses, and raw honey.

Coffee and Tea Brewed from roasted coffee beans, coffee is generally acceptable on the Paleo diet, as is tea. Both should be consumed in small quantities, without adding milk or non-Paleo sweeteners.

Dark Chocolate Dark chocolate (70 percent or higher), cacao, and carob are types of chocolate generally accepted as Paleo. They come in multiple forms, including chips and powder. Avoid chocolate with added ingredients, including sugar. You may also be able to find Paleo-certified chocolate products from brands such as Enjoy Life and Hu Kitchen.

CONTINUED

Off the Table

Alcohol While alcohol is not considered Paleo friendly, many Paleo eaters enjoy grain-free spirits and alcohols made from fruit, such as wine and tequila, in moderation. Ultimately, the key is to limit sugars and watch your body's responses to figure out what works for you.

Beans and Legumes While beans and legumes are generally considered to be a "healthy" food, they contain phytic acid. Because this acid binds to nutrients in food, it prevents you from absorbing them, making legumes nutrient-deficient and to be avoided. Legumes include beans, peanuts, soy, and peas.

Cured Meats Cured meats, such as ham, salami, prosciutto, and sausage, are processed and laden with additives and preservatives. However, meats such as bacon labeled "no added nitrates or nitrites" are made with celery juice and can be consumed on a Paleo diet.

Dairy Cow's milk, goat milk, and dairy products made from animal milk are not Paleo friendly. Fortunately, almond milk, coconut milk, and others make great substitutes.

Fats Cooking fats derived from foods that are off-limits, including canola oil, corn oil, and peanut oil are not Paleo friendly and should be avoided.

Grains The Paleo diet is grain- and gluten-free, meaning barely, corn, oats, quinoa, rice, rye, and wheat are off-limits.

Processed Foods Processed foods provide minimal nutritional value and should be avoided on the Paleo diet.

Refined Sugar Refined sugars such as aspartame, brown sugar, cane sugar, and artificial sweeteners are off-limits.

The Power of Paleo Meal Prep

When it comes to following the Paleo diet, there's one strategy that works time and again: planning ahead. Because when do we most often throw our diet out the window? When we're busy!

The most important part of Paleo meal prep is planning and blocking out time for cooking. What if I told you that you could meal prep a week of Paleo meals on Sunday to keep you out of the kitchen all week long? Yep, that's the beauty of meal prep.

Most important, meal prepping means you will have delicious Paleo breakfasts, lunches, and dinners ready to go so you avoid the temptation of unhealthy quick and easy choices.

My favorite trick when preparing meals in advance is to double the recipe. By making an extra batch of food, you'll have enough for a meal the next day, or you can freeze the second batch for another time. These freezer meals will taste good and make you feel good, saving the day when you are truly busy beyond belief. A few of my favorite freezer-friendly meals include Beef Chili (page 28), Short Rib and Root Veggie Stew (page 132) and of course, my Sweet Potato Chicken Nuggets and Parsnip Fries (page 120).

Meal Prep 101

If you are new to meal prep, don't let it intimidate you. I promise this way of life will save you so much potential stress throughout the week. My biggest piece of advice is to sit down and plan before you actually start cooking. Remember to be patient and find your rhythm while multitasking in the kitchen. The more you cook multiple things at once, the better you will get at it. The following is an outline of the key steps in the meal prep process.

Planning

No matter how long you have been eating Paleo, planning and prepping for the week ahead will always work to your benefit in the long run. Meal prep shouldn't be stressful; it's actually quite simple if you take time to plan.

Throughout the following chapter you will find three meal plans (two weeks each), shopping lists, and recipes to guide you on this journey, but it is just that—a guide. Feel free to swap in recipes from other chapters of the book based on what you want to eat each week. After all, if you aren't excited by a recipe, you aren't going to eat the meal you have prepped. Keep in mind that these meal plans are designed to make your work week easier and do not include weekends.

When planning, make a grocery list and purchase only the foods you need. You will also want to do an inventory of your pantry and spice rack every once in a while to avoid running out of the essentials. Keeping a running list on the refrigerator or taking a photo of your refrigerator, freezer, and pantry on your phone before you head to the grocery store might make this easier. The point is to find a system that works best for you and stick to it.

Ingredient Reuse

Meal prep plans that use and reuse ingredients smartly help save time and money. That's what the meal plans in this book will do. As you begin building your own meal prep plans with the bonus recipes in this book, be sure to use recipes that call for similar ingredients and staples in a variety of meals. For example, choose recipes that use staples like cauliflower rice and cauliflower mash, or stretch an ingredient, like cilantro or coconut milk, across more than one recipe.

Spice Things Up

With an endless list of spices, eating Paleo should never be boring. That is why no Paleo pantry is complete without a growing spice rack.

In addition to adding flavor to your favorite Paleo dishes, a number of common herbs and spices also offer several health benefits. In fact, some have shown to possess high levels of antioxidant activity, while others help protect against chronic conditions.

Get the most from your herbs and spices (both in flavor and health benefits) by storing them in airtight containers away from heat, moisture, and direct sunlight, and by using them before their sell-by dates.

The following are some of my favorites that I use across many of my recipes. If you don't already have these spices, you don't need to buy them all at once. Plan to pick up a few each time you go to the market.

Basil, in both its fresh and dried form, is used to add flavor to a variety of dishes throughout this book. Basil is traditionally used in Italian and Mediterranean recipes. Basil can provide macronutrients and a range of antioxidants.

Cinnamon has been shown to lower inflammation and reduce blood glucose levels. Cinnamon is an aromatic spice that is used in a wide variety of cuisines and adds warmth and depth of flavor to both sweet and savory dishes.

Chili powder is made by grinding dry chile peppers and adding a variety of other spices to create a blend. The exact blend varies by brand. Chili powder has been linked to a boost in fat-burning capacity.

Cumin is commonly used in a variety of cuisines, including Latin American, Middle Eastern, North African, and Indian, and is often used in spice blends, such as garam masala, curry powder, and adobos. Cumin is a rich source of iron and promotes digestion.

Oregano is an aromatic herb that can be used in fresh or dried form. Often used in Mediterranean and Mexican cuisine, it is also a common component of spice blends like chili powder and Italian seasoning. Oregano is also rich in antioxidants and can reduce inflammation.

Paprika is made from a variety of dried red peppers. There are three varieties ranging from sweet and mild to bitter and hot: sweet paprika, hot paprika, and smoked paprika. Paprika is high in vitamin C.

Turmeric is an anti-inflammatory and antioxidant. This spice is responsible for giving curry its rich gold color and is commonly found in other Asian dishes.

Cooking and Prep

Now that you have planned and purchased ingredients for your recipes, the next step is the meal prep. You will want to set aside a few hours over the weekend or on a free day to do all of the prep and cooking. While this may sound intimidating, dedicating this time over the weekend will set you up for success during the week ahead.

The meal prep plans and the recipes throughout this book will guide you through this process with tips and tricks for managing multiple tasks in the kitchen, speeding up prep, and more!

While the cooking may seem like a chore, keep it fun. Make it a family affair, invite friends over to do their meal prep, or listen to a podcast or audiobook as you prep and cook.

Containers and Equipment

Good-quality containers are essential for keeping your food fresh as long as possible. In our house we use glass containers for many reasons. Although glass is a little more of an investment than plastic, they are more durable, and you can easily see what is inside. It is important to have containers you like in multiple sizes and shapes to portion your food. I like to use sectioned containers with multiple compartments, round containers, and even mason jars, depending on what meal I'm storing. To help you get started, I have included storage container recommendations for each of the meal plans in the book.

Here are some other things to look for when buying containers for meal prepping:

BPA-free BPA stands for bisphenol A, which is a chemical found in plastics like food containers and water bottles. Research has shown that BPA can seep into food or beverages from plastic containers made of BPA. Given the negative effects of BPA, it is important to look for containers that are BPA-free. This is another reason I opt for glass storage containers.

Stackable Space has been and always will be at a premium, especially in the kitchen. After all, I know we all have a cupboard or a drawer packed full of storage containers and lids. When you make meal prep a part of your regular routine, you will need to upgrade the forgotten drawer of mismatched containers. I recommend opting for containers that are stackable to keep your cupboard or drawers organized and manageable.

Freezer-safe There will be times when you prep and have more than you need for the week. That's when having containers that are freezer-safe is key. As I recommended earlier in the book, you may also double recipes and keep them in the freezer for future use.

Microwave-safe Many of the meals throughout this book recommend reheating in the microwave as this will be most convenient. Be sure to choose containers that you can use in the microwave. Oven-safe is an added bonus.

Dishwasher-safe This one is pretty straightforward: Opt for containers that you can put in the dishwasher, and cleanup will be a breeze.

Here's a secret: You don't need to have a kitchen full of fancy equipment to be a meal prep pro. In addition to a variety of storage containers, all you need to get started are a handful of basic kitchen tools:

- Aluminum foil
- Baking sheets
- Chef's knife
- Cutting board
- Food processor and/or high-speed blender
- Glass baking dishes
- Measuring cups and spoons
- Mixing bowls
- Muffin tins
- Parchment paper
- Pots and pans
- Pressure cooker and/or slow cooker
- Whisk, spatula, tongs, mixing spoon
- Wire cooling rack

Storage and Labeling

Labeling your meals, especially those going into the freezer, is important to make sure you know what you have and when it needs to be used by. I recommend keeping tape and a permanent marker near the refrigerator so that you can write the name of the dish and use by date when the meal goes in the refrigerator or freezer.

After labeling your meals, store them so that you can grab and go. I like to place the foods that I need to eat first in the front at eye level.

Thawing and Reheating

Most of the recipes in each of the meal prep plans throughout the book go in the refrigerator for the week, and I have included instructions with each recipe on how to reheat. Microwaving is the most convenient and quickest way to reheat food. I recommend reheating in one-minute intervals and keeping a close eye on your meal, stirring occasionally for an even temperature throughout. You can also reheat your meals using the oven or stovetop.

When reheating leftovers, look for an internal temperature of 165°F. For leftovers that are frozen, it is important to thaw first and then reheat. The best way to defrost frozen food is to place the frozen item in the refrigerator to thaw. This requires giving yourself enough time to have it thawed before you are ready to enjoy it. For example, before I head to work in the morning, I'll pull out dinner from the freezer and place it in the refrigerator to defrost before I get home in the evening.

If you did not plan ahead, the cold-water thawing method can be quicker than defrosting in the refrigerator, but requires more attention. The food must be in a leakproof container and submerged in cold water. Replace the water every 30 minutes until thawed.

FOOD STORAGE

The good news is most Paleo ingredients prep perfectly and freeze well, too. When purchasing and prepping food, it is important to know how long it can be stored in the refrigerator and freezer. Remember that this a guideline, so always use your best judgement as some preparations store better than others. I have also included special storage tips within each recipe.

	FOODS	REFRIGERATOR	FREEZER
FRESH PROTEINS	Eggs	3 to 5 weeks	Does not freeze well
	Fish	1 to 2 days	1 month
	Poultry	1 to 2 days	9 to 12 months
	Beef, Pork, Lamb	1 to 2 days	3 to 4 months
	Bacon	7 days	1 month
COOKED PROTEINS	Eggs	3 to 5 days	Does not freeze well
	Fish	up to 3 days	1 month
	Poultry	3 to 5 days	2 to 4 months
	Beef, Pork, Lamb	3 to 5 days	3 to 6 months
	Bacon	7 days	1 month

The Meal Prep Plans

Now that you understand the basics of meal prep and the Paleo diet, it's time to put everything you've read into practice. To help you out along the way, I've designed three, two-week meal plans built from recipes that store and reheat well.

These meal plans are intended to support different goals and lifestyles and are jumping-off points for maintaining a Paleo diet with meal prep.

New to Paleo: This is the ideal plan if you are new to the Paleo diet and are looking to simplify your transition through meal prep. You will find that the recipes in this plan are the simplest and most straightforward, and use many ingredients you likely already have on hand.

The Athlete: This is a performance-based meal prep plan designed to support the nutritional needs of active Paleo eaters who regularly work out or train. The breakfast, lunch, and dinner recipes throughout this plan focus on meals with higher calories, more carbs, proteins, and macronutrients. While I have not included snacks in each plan, feel free to add snacks from chapter 8 as needed to supplement your intake needs and goals. Just be sure to adjust your shopping list and prep as needed.

Paleo as a Lifestyle: This meal prep plan was designed to make it as easy as possible to continue to reap the benefits of the diet while getting meal prep inspiration. As with the other plans in this book, this prep will offer breakfast, lunch, and dinner options. The recipes are a bit more creative and fun to keep you from getting bored with traditional Paleo.

The plan for each week supports a typical five-day work week. If you want to meal prep enough food for the full week, I recommend doubling up on a recipe or two that will freeze well or using the bonus recipes in Part 3 (page 87) to cook on the weekends.

These meal plans are meant to be flexible, so if a particular recipe doesn't appeal to you, you can easily swap it out for one of the recipes in the back of the book. You can also add snacks to any of the meal plans, should you desire to. Just be sure to update your grocery list so that you have everything you need.

About the Recipes

The meal prep plans ahead are filled with simple yet delicious Paleo recipes that are ideal for meal prepping. You will find recipes for breakfast, lunch, and dinner that can be made in advance and reheated to enjoy any night of the week. In addition to the recipes throughout the Paleo meal prep plans, I've included bonus breakfast, lunch, and dinner recipes in the back of the book that are not included in the meal plans. These recipes can be used to create and build your own meal plans or to swap in for recipes in the meal plans provided. Furthermore, I have included a chapter of staple recipes where you will find various Paleo sauces, condiments, and other staples that will be used across the meal plans and recipes in this book. There is also a snack chapter packed full of my favorite Paleo snacks that you can prep to enjoy throughout the week in addition to breakfast, lunch, and dinner.

Although I've divided these recipes into breakfast, lunch, and dinner, there are no rules as to when you eat what. Feel free to enjoy your breakfast casserole for dinner or your chicken and veggies for breakfast. All of the recipes throughout the book are tasty; filling; and free of added sugar, grains, dairy, and legumes. They are Paleo meal prep staples in my house, and I'm sure they will quickly become favorites in yours as well.

As you begin, remember to read through each recipe and meal plan completely, and gather all of the ingredients and kitchen tools you will need in advance. I also suggest that you follow each recipe exactly as written your first time trying it. Then, as you become more comfortable in the kitchen using these ingredients, you can switch things up. Throughout the recipes, you will also see that I have included helpful tips and suggestions for ingredient substitutes, cooking hacks, and my recommendations for smart shopping. Finally, most of the recipes make three to five servings, perfect for prepping for the week, but pay attention to the serving size so you can plan your grocery list properly. The meal plans are developed for one person but can be easily doubled as needed if you are prepping for two people.

Ready, set—time to go meal prep!

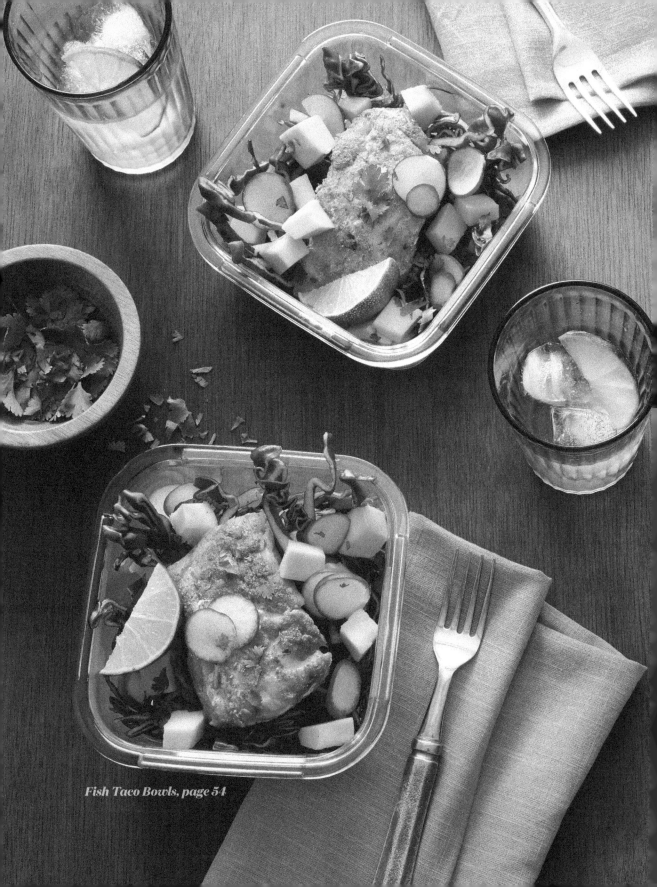

Fish Taco Bowls, page 54

The Meal Prep Plans

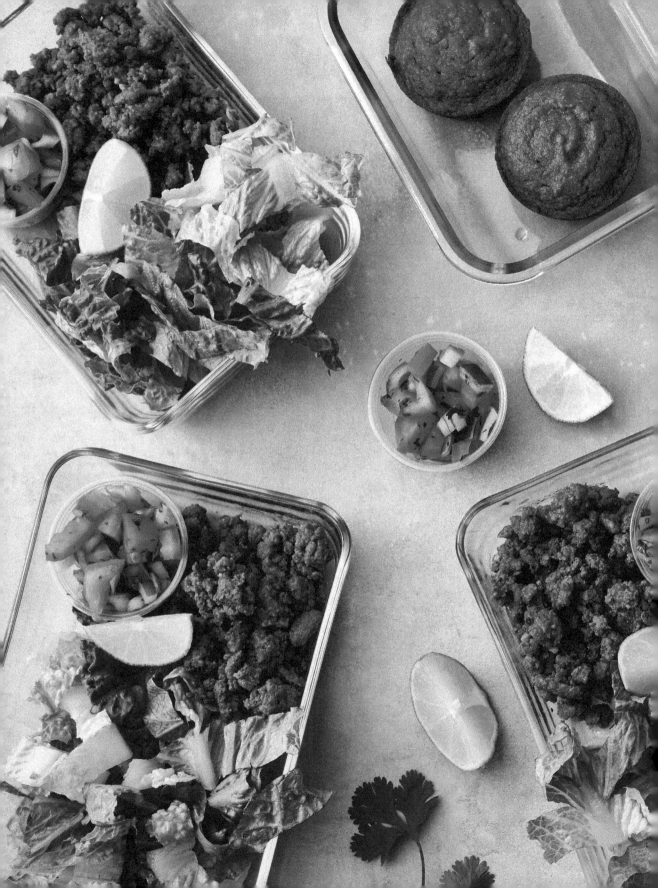

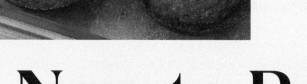

New to Paleo

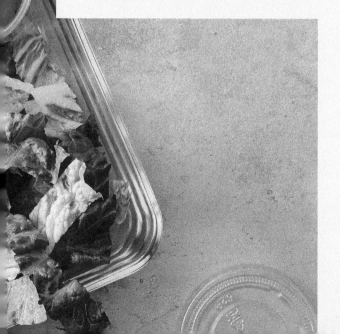

This meal prep plan was designed specifically for Paleo newbies to kick-start your Paleo adventure. The perfect plan for beginners, this prep includes breakfast, lunch, and dinner recipes that are ideal for those new to the Paleo lifestyle. You will find that this is the easiest meal plan in the book with the simplest, most straightforward recipes—without lacking in flavor. In fact, in this plan I have snuck in my favorite meal prep hack: Double the prep and freeze half the batch for the following week. By following this hack for the Beef Chili (page 28), you will do the prep in week one but eat it throughout both weeks, saving you even more time.

The recipes in this prep use ingredients that you likely already have on hand, even if this is your first foray into Paleo, so you can enjoy comfort food favorites like Spaghetti Squash and Meatballs (page 36), and takeout favorites like Taco Salad (page 31) and Chicken and Broccoli Stir-Fry (page 41). Whether you are looking to improve your health or spend less time in the kitchen, this plan can help you accomplish your goals.

WEEK ONE

	BREAKFAST	LUNCH	DINNER
MONDAY	Mixed Veggie Baked Egg Cups (page 25)	Taco Salad (page 31)	Beef Chili (page 28)
TUESDAY	*Leftover* Mixed Veggie Baked Egg Cups	*Leftover* Taco Salad	Sheet Pan Garlic and Herb Chicken and Veggies (page 27)
WEDNESDAY	*Leftover* Mixed Veggie Baked Egg Cups	*Leftover* Beef Chili	*Leftover* Taco Salad
THURSDAY	*Leftover* Mixed Veggie Baked Egg Cups	*Leftover* Taco Salad	*Leftover* Sheet Pan Garlic and Herb Chicken and Veggies
FRIDAY	*Leftover* Mixed Veggie Baked Egg Cups	*Leftover* Sheet Pan Garlic and Herb Chicken and Veggies	*Leftover* Beef Chili

Shopping List

Pantry

- Basil, dried
- Black pepper, freshly ground
- Chicken broth
- Chili powder
- Cumin
- Garlic salt
- Milk, unsweetened almond
- Oil, coconut
- Oil, extra-virgin olive
- Onion powder
- Oregano, dried
- Paprika
- Red pepper flakes
- Sea salt
- Tomatoes, crushed, 1 (28-ounce) can
- Tomatoes, diced, 1 (14.5-ounce) can
- Tomato paste

Produce

- Basil (1 bunch)
- Bell pepper, green (2)
- Broccoli (1 head)
- Cilantro (1 bunch)
- Garlic (2 heads)
- Lettuce, romaine (1 large head)
- Limes (2)
- Mushrooms, Baby Bella (1 small container)
- Onion, red (1)
- Onion, white (2)
- Parsley (1 bunch)
- Spinach, 1 (10-ounce) bag
- Squash, yellow (1)
- Tomato (1)
- Tomato, plum (1)

Protein

- Boneless chicken breast (1 pound)
- Eggs (1 dozen)
- Ground beef (3 pounds)

Equipment List

- Baking sheet
- Chef's knife
- Cutting board
- Measuring cups and spoons
- Mixing bowls
- Mixing spoon
- Muffin tin
- Pressure cooker or slow cooker
- Skillet
- Tongs
- Whisk

Storage Containers

Mixed Veggie Baked Egg Cups: 5 (24-ounce) single-compartment meal prep containers

Sheet Pan Garlic and Herb Chicken and Veggies: 3 (24-ounce) single-compartment meal prep containers

Beef Chili: 6 (24-ounce) single-compartment meal prep containers

Taco Salad: 4 (24-ounce) single-compartment meal prep containers, 4 (2-ounce) sauce cups, and 4 small plastic sandwich bags

Step-by-Step Prep

1. Prepare the Mixed Veggie Baked Egg Cups (page 25) through step 5.

2. While the egg cups are cooking, prepare steps 2 and 3 of the Sheet Pan Garlic and Herb Chicken and Veggies (page 27).

3. When the egg cups are finished cooking, remove from oven and raise the oven temperature to 450°F. Roast the Sheet Pan Garlic and Herb Chicken and Veggies according to step 4.

4. While the chicken and vegetables are cooking, prepare the Beef Chili (page 28) through step 5.

5. While the chili cooks, prepare the Taco Salad (page 31) in full.

6. Remove the chicken and vegetables from the oven and complete step 5 of the Sheet Pan Garlic and Herb Chicken and Veggies.

7. Complete steps 6 and 7 of the Beef Chili and step 6 of the Mixed Veggie Baked Egg Cups.

8. When the food is cool, close and store the containers in the refrigerator, reserving half of the Beef Chili in the freezer.

Mixed Veggie Baked Egg Cups

Serves 5 — Prep time: 10 minutes — Cook time: 25 minutes

These baked egg cups have been a staple in my meal prep repertoire for years. This recipe is perfectly portioned and easy to prep thanks to a handy muffin tin. Perhaps most important, you can customize this recipe based on the vegetables you have in the refrigerator. Just be sure to opt for veggies and greens that are not water dense so that the egg cups stay together and do not get runny. If two egg cups are not enough to fill you up, serve with half an avocado or half a baked sweet potato.

Coconut oil, for greasing

2 cups spinach, chopped

1 large tomato, seeds removed and diced

½ cup Baby Bella mushrooms, diced

10 eggs

¼ cup unsweetened almond milk

½ teaspoon sea salt

Freshly ground black pepper

1. Preheat the oven to 350°F.
2. Grease 10 cups of a muffin tin with coconut oil.
3. Divide the spinach, tomatoes, and mushrooms evenly between the 10 cups of the tin.
4. In a large bowl, whisk together the eggs, almond milk, and salt, and season with pepper. Fill each cup about three-quarters full with the egg mixture, pouring over the veggies already in each.
5. Bake for 25 minutes, until the eggs are set and puff up in the tin.
6. Let the cups cool for a few minutes, then run a butter knife around the edges of each cup and remove. Divide the egg cups between 5 containers.

CONTINUED

Mixed Veggie Baked Egg Cups

CONTINUED

STORAGE: Once cooled, store in covered containers in the refrigerator for up to 5 days or freeze for up to 2 months. Reheat refrigerated egg cups in the microwave for 25 to 30 seconds, or 50 to 60 seconds if frozen. You can also heat these in 15-second increments to be sure they retain the right texture.

SIMPLE SWAP: Use this recipe as the base for an endless number of variations. Swap in jalapeño peppers, bell peppers, onions, or even ground sausage. Look for nitrate-free sausage, or make your own using one of the sausage recipes found throughout this book.

Per Serving (2 Egg Cups): Calories: 177; Fat: 12g; Protein: 12g; Total Carbs: 4g; Fiber: 1g; Sodium: 366mg; Iron: 2g

Sheet Pan Garlic and Herb Chicken and Veggies

Serves 3 — Prep time: 10 minutes — Cook time: 25 minutes

Perhaps the most important cooking technique to master when learning to meal prep is the perfect sheet pan meal—and it's easier than you think. Pick a protein, choose your veggies, add a marinade, and voilà! The best part is you can customize this recipe if you have any vegetables left over from the week before. Forgot to eat those bell pepper slices you prepped for a snack? Have some leftover carrot sticks or broccoli florets? Simply add them to the pan.

2 tablespoons extra-virgin olive oil

2 garlic cloves, minced

2 tablespoons parsley

1 tablespoon freshly squeezed lime juice

Sea salt

Freshly ground black pepper

1 pound boneless skinless chicken breast, chopped into 1-inch pieces

1 head broccoli, trimmed into florets

1 large yellow squash, chopped

1 medium onion, chopped

1. Preheat the oven to 450°F.

2. In a medium bowl, whisk together the olive oil, garlic, parsley, and lime juice. Season with salt and pepper.

3. On a baking sheet, arrange the chicken, broccoli, squash, and onion. Drizzle with the garlic and herb mixture and toss with tongs until all the chicken and veggies are coated.

4. Bake for 20 to 25 minutes, until the chicken and veggies are cooked through. Chicken is cooked when it reaches an internal temperature of 165°F.

5. Divide the chicken and vegetables between three containers.

STORAGE: Once cooled, store in covered containers in the refrigerator for up to 5 days. To reheat, microwave for 1 to 2 minutes, or bake in a 400°F oven for 8 to 10 minutes.

SIMPLE SWAP: If you do not have parsley in the pantry, opt for dried basil or oregano. You can also try swapping out the garlic and herb marinade for another marinade or dressing of your choice.

Per Serving (1 container): Calories: 367; Fat: 14g; Protein: 42g; Total Carbs: 22g; Fiber: 7g; Sodium: 192mg; Iron: 3g

Beef Chili

Serves 6 — Prep time: 10 minutes — Cook time: 20 minutes

There is no better comfort food when the chill of fall sets in than a big bowl of chili. While chili can be quite the production and require a lot of ingredients and hours in the kitchen, this recipe is built on 10 simple ingredients and can be made in just 30 minutes. But don't let the simplicity of this recipe fool you. It is still packed with all of the warm, bold flavors of a chili that has been simmering for hours on the stove thanks to the pressure cooker.

3 tablespoons extra-virgin olive oil

2 pounds ground beef

2 teaspoons sea salt, divided

2 large onions, diced

2 green bell peppers, seeded and diced

6 garlic cloves, finely grated or minced

4 tablespoons chili powder

1 teaspoon ground cumin

2 teaspoons dried oregano

3 (8-ounce) cans diced tomatoes

½ cup chicken broth

1. Set the sauté setting on a pressure cooker to high. Put the oil in the cooking pot and allow it to heat up.

2. Add the beef to the cooking pot and season with 1 teaspoon of salt. Cook for about 5 minutes, stirring occasionally until brown. Transfer browned beef to a plate.

3. Add the onions, bell peppers, and garlic to the cooking pot. Season with the remaining salt and cook until softened, about 5 minutes.

4. Add the chili powder and cumin and cook until fragrant, about 1 minute.

5. Return the beef to the cooking pot. Add the oregano, diced tomatoes, and chicken broth. Cover the pressure cooker and cook on high for 8 minutes. Once cooking is complete, let pressure release naturally.

6. Carefully remove the lid and stir the chili.

7. Divide the chili evenly between 6 containers.

STORAGE: Once cooled, store in covered containers in the refrigerator for up to 5 days. Store in freezer-safe containers for up to 2 months. To reheat refrigerated chili, microwave uncovered for 2 to 3 minutes. To defrost, refrigerate overnight and microwave uncovered for 2 to 3 minutes.

COOKING HACK: If you do not have a pressure cooker, you can make this recipe in a slow cooker. Cook on high for 3 to 4 hours or on low for 6 to 8 hours. If your slow cooker does not have a sauté setting, complete steps 1 through 4 on the stovetop.

Per Serving (1 container): Calories: 428; Fat: 21g; Protein: 44g; Total Carbs: 15g; Fiber: 4g; Sodium: 1053mg; Iron: 6g

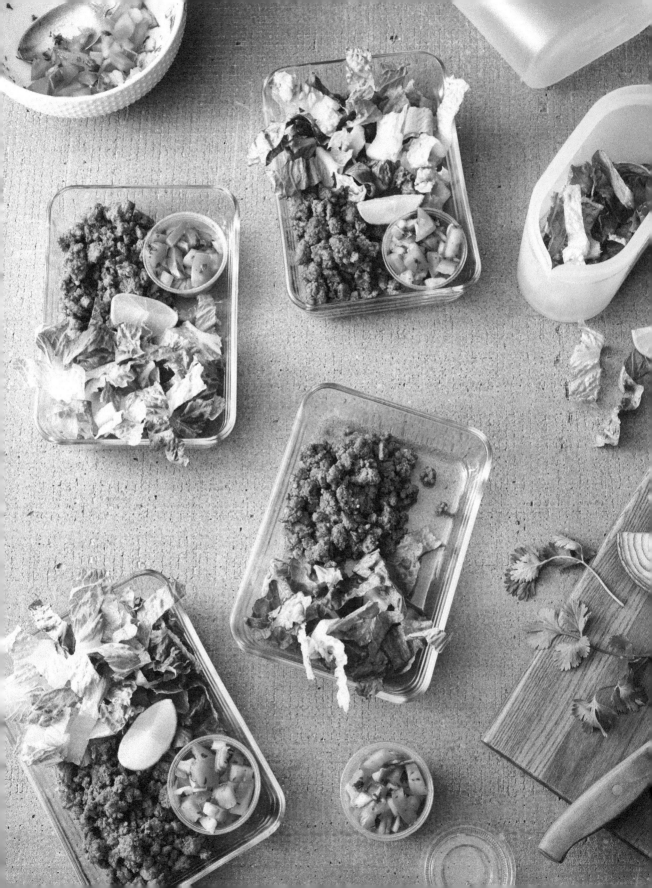

Taco Salad

Serves 4 — Prep time: 15 minutes — Cook time: 10 minutes

When I think of the perfect prep-ahead recipe, taco salad is front and center. Not only is this recipe easy to prep in advance, but the flavors in the taco seasoning marinate together even more overnight. An added bonus is that it's fun to put together when the time comes to dig in. Simply remove the lettuce, pico de gallo, and lime wedge from the container when reheating the beef, and then toss it all together for the perfect taco salad.

1 tablespoon extra-virgin olive oil

1 pound ground beef

2 tablespoons Taco Seasoning (page 92)

½ cup water

1 plum tomato, diced

¼ red onion, finely diced

1 lime, divided in half lengthwise

Sea salt

1 tablespoon cilantro, finely chopped

4 cups shredded romaine lettuce

1. Prepare the taco seasoning and set aside.

2. In a large skillet, heat the oil over medium-high heat.

3. Add the ground beef and cook about 5 minutes, until the beef starts to brown. Drain the excess fat. Add the taco seasoning and the water.

4. Lower the heat to medium-low and let simmer for another 3 to 5 minutes, until thickened.

5. Meanwhile, in a small bowl combine the tomatoes, onion, and the juice of ½ of a lime. Season with salt. Add the cilantro and stir until well combined.

6. Divide the romaine lettuce into 4 small sandwich bags.

7. Divide the pico de gallo into 4 2-ounce cups with lids.

8. Slice the remaining half of the lime into 4 wedges.

9. Divide the beef, romaine lettuce, pico de gallo, and lime wedges into 4 containers.

CONTINUED

Taco Salad

CONTINUED

STORAGE: Once cooled, store in covered containers in the refrigerator for up to 5 days. To reheat, remove the romaine lettuce, pico de gallo, and lime wedge from the container and microwave the ground beef for 1 to 2 minutes. Assemble salads and enjoy!

SIMPLE SWAP: Switch things up and swap ground chicken, pork, or turkey for the ground beef in this recipe. To keep the tacos succulent but not oily, I recommend opting for 90% lean ground meat.

Per Serving (1 container): Calories: 280; Fat: 14g; Protein: 33g; Total Carbs: 6g; Fiber: 2g; Sodium: 238mg; Iron: 5g

	BREAKFAST	LUNCH	DINNER
MONDAY	Sweet Potato Cinnamon Muffins (page 39)	Chicken and Broccoli Stir-Fry (page 41)	Spaghetti Squash and Meatballs (page 36)
TUESDAY	*Leftover* Sweet Potato Cinnamon Muffins	*Leftover* Chicken and Broccoli Stir-Fry	*Leftover* Beef Chili
WEDNESDAY	*Leftover* Sweet Potato Cinnamon Muffins	*Leftover* Spaghetti Squash and Meatballs	*Leftover* Chicken and Broccoli Stir-Fry
THURSDAY	*Leftover* Sweet Potato Cinnamon Muffins	*Leftover* Chicken and Broccoli Stir-Fry	*Leftover* Beef Chili
FRIDAY	*Leftover* Sweet Potato Cinnamon Muffins	*Leftover* Beef Chili	*Leftover* Spaghetti Squash and Meatballs

Shopping List

Pantry

- ☐ Baking soda
- ☐ Basil, dried
- ☐ Black pepper
- ☐ Coconut aminos
- ☐ Flour, almond
- ☐ Flour, coconut
- ☐ Flour, tapioca
- ☐ Garlic powder
- ☐ Ground cinnamon
- ☐ Maple syrup
- ☐ Oil, coconut
- ☐ Oil, olive
- ☐ Oil, sesame
- ☐ Onion powder
- ☐ Oregano, dried
- ☐ Red pepper flakes
- ☐ Sea salt
- ☐ Sweet potato puree (1 can)
- ☐ Tomatoes, crushed, 1 (28-ounce) can
- ☐ Tomato paste
- ☐ Vinegar, apple cider

Produce

- ☐ Basil (1 bunch)
- ☐ Broccoli (1 head)
- ☐ Garlic (2 heads)
- ☐ Ginger (1 small piece)
- ☐ Onion, white (1)
- ☐ Pepper, red bell (2)
- ☐ Squash, spaghetti (1)

Protein

- ☐ Boneless chicken breast (1 pound)
- ☐ Eggs (4)
- ☐ Ground beef (8 ounces)

Equipment List

- ☐ Aluminum foil
- ☐ Baking sheets
- ☐ Chef's knife
- ☐ Cutting board
- ☐ Large pot
- ☐ Measuring cups and spoons
- ☐ Mixing bowls
- ☐ Muffin tin
- ☐ Skillet
- ☐ Spatula
- ☐ Tongs
- ☐ Whisk
- ☐ Wire cooling rack

Storage Containers

Spaghetti Squash and Meatballs: 3 (24-ounce) single-compartment meal prep containers

Sweet Potato Cinnamon Muffins: 5 (24-ounce) single-compartment meal prep containers

Chicken and Broccoli Stir-Fry: 4 (24-ounce) single-compartment meal prep containers

Step-by-Step Prep

1. Prepare the Spaghetti Squash and Meatballs (page 36) through step 8.

2. While the meatballs cook, prepare the Sweet Potato Cinnamon Muffins (page 39) through step 5.

3. Remove the meatballs from the oven when done and lower the oven temperature to 350°F. Place the muffins in the oven and complete step 9 of Spaghetti Squash and Meatballs.

4. Prepare the Chicken and Broccoli Stir-Fry (page 41) in full.

5. Complete step 7 of Sweet Potato Cinnamon Muffins.

6. Remove Beef Chili from the freezer and put it in the refrigerator to thaw.

7. When the food is cool, close containers and store in the refrigerator.

Spaghetti Squash and Meatballs

Serves 3 — Prep time: 40 minutes — Cook time: 1 hour 20 minutes

This recipe is a low-carb, veggie-loaded version of one of my all-time favorite recipes: spaghetti and meatballs. If you have never worked with spaghetti squash, simply follow this recipe. I have broken down the instructions for the perfect al dente spaghetti squash. It is important the squash is al dente because you will be reheating the dish in the microwave during the week, and you don't want the "spaghetti" to get soggy. Once you have mastered this recipe, you can use spaghetti squash in place of pasta in a number of your favorite dishes; try it with Pesto Sauce (page 94)—or in place of the noodles in lasagna.

1 small spaghetti squash

8 ounces ground beef

1 egg yolk

2 tablespoons almond flour

¼ teaspoon dried oregano

¼ teaspoon onion powder

¼ teaspoon garlic powder

¼ teaspoon sea salt

¼ teaspoon freshly ground black pepper

1 cup Marinara Sauce (page 93)

1. Preheat the oven to 425°F.

2. While the oven heats, halve the spaghetti squash lengthwise. Using a large spoon, scrape out all the seeds and loose fibers from each half.

3. Line a baking sheet with aluminum foil. Place the spaghetti squash face down on the baking sheet and bake for 50 minutes.

4. While the squash is cooking, in a large bowl, combine the ground beef, egg yolk, almond flour, oregano, onion powder, garlic powder, salt, and pepper.

5. Form the ground beef mixture into meatballs and put them on an aluminum foil–lined baking sheet. Put the sheet in the refrigerator until the meatballs are ready to cook.

6. Prepare the marinara sauce and set aside.

7. Remove the squash from the oven and turn the halves over so they are faceup. Allow them to cool for 5 minutes, then scrape the insides of the squash halves with a fork to create "spaghetti" strands.

8. While the squash is cooling, raise the oven temperature to 450°F. Put the baking sheet with the meatballs in the oven and bake for about 30 minutes, until cooked through.

9. Divide the spaghetti and meatballs between 3 containers. Top with ⅓ cup of marinara sauce each.

STORAGE: Once cooled, store in covered containers in the refrigerator for up to 5 days. To reheat, microwave for 2 to 3 minutes.

SMART SHOPPING: While I do my best to make most ingredients from scratch each week, sometimes I opt for a little shortcut. If you prefer to purchase a pre-made marinara sauce, look for a version with no added sugar. We always keep a jar of Rao's or Victoria in the pantry just in case.

Per Serving (1 container): Calories: 384; Fat: 12g; Protein: 28g; Total Carbs: 48g; Fiber: 11g; Sodium: 647mg; Iron: 6g

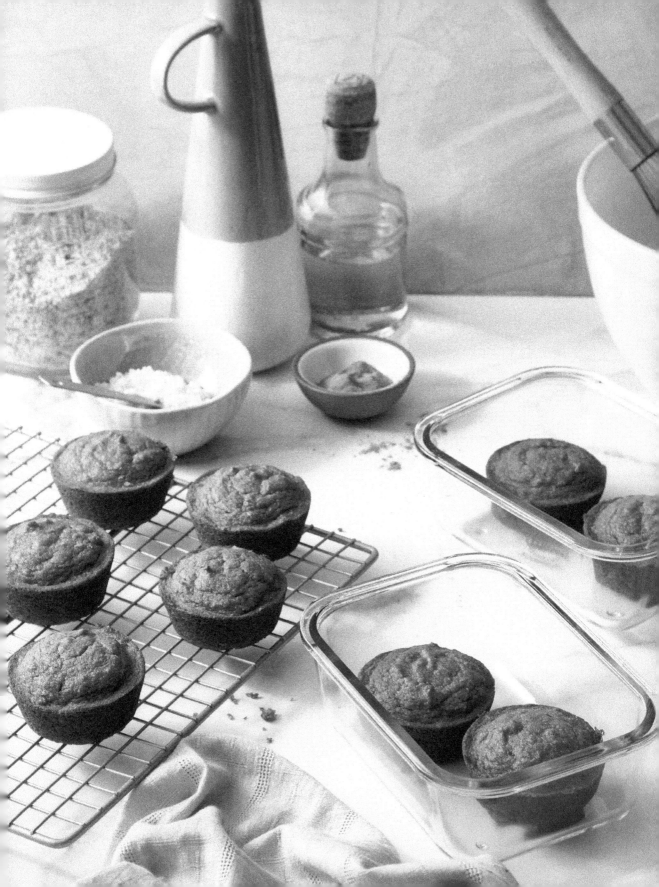

Sweet Potato Cinnamon Muffins

Serves 5 — Prep time: 10 minutes — Cook time: 20 minutes

Muffins are one of my favorite breakfast options to prep in advance, but the challenge is filling the muffins with goodness and not just empty calories. I have developed a number of muffin recipes that are filled with fruits for natural sweetness, but in this recipe the sweet potato gives these muffins their moist texture. Meanwhile, the cinnamon and maple syrup come together for a warm, sweet finish. Enjoy right from the refrigerator, warmed in the microwave, or lightly toasted with a little ghee.

4 tablespoons coconut oil, room temp, divided

3 large eggs

½ cup sweet potato puree

3 tablespoons pure maple syrup

1 tablespoon apple cider vinegar

1¼ cups almond flour

3 tablespoons coconut flour

¼ cup tapioca flour

1 teaspoon baking soda

2 teaspoons cinnamon

¼ teaspoon sea salt

1. Preheat the oven to 350°F.
2. While the oven heats, grease 10 cups of a muffin tin with 1 tablespoon coconut oil.
3. In a large bowl, whisk together the eggs, sweet potato puree, maple syrup, the remaining coconut oil, and apple cider vinegar.
4. In a separate bowl, combine the almond flour, coconut flour, tapioca flour, baking soda, cinnamon, and sea salt.
5. Slowly add the dry ingredients to the wet ingredients until just combined. Divide the mixture evenly between the 10 greased cups in the tin.
6. Bake for 20 minutes, or until a toothpick inserted in the center comes out clean.
7. Transfer to a wire rack to cool completely. Then divide between 5 containers.

CONTINUED

Sweet Potato Cinnamon Muffins

CONTINUED

STORAGE: Store in covered containers in the refrigerator for up to 5 days.

SMART SHOPPING: Tapioca flour is a starch extracted from the cassava plant and is a common Paleo alternative to corn starch. It is typically found in the baking aisle near the gluten-free flours. Bob's Red Mill is a common brand that I like to use.

COOKING HACK: Instead of using a canned sweet potato puree, make your own. Bake a sweet potato at 425°F for 1 hour. Let cool and then remove the skin and mash the sweet potato flesh. Squeeze gently with a paper towel to remove excess water.

Per Serving (2 muffins): Calories: 268; Fat: 15g; Protein: 6g; Total Carbs: 26g; Fiber: 3g; Sodium: 483mg; Iron: 1g

Chicken and Broccoli Stir-Fry

Serves 4 — Prep time: 10 minutes — Cook time: 10 minutes

One of the easiest ways to keep meal prep recipes exciting throughout the week is to opt for recipes that taste like a guilty pleasure. This stir-fry is a great, healthy alternative to takeout because it is made from whole, flavorful ingredients. And because all the hard work is done in advance, it is faster to heat up than ordering delivery!

2 tablespoons sesame oil

1 onion, diced

1 tablespoon minced garlic

1 tablespoon minced ginger

1 pound boneless chicken breast, diced

¼ cup coconut aminos

1 head broccoli, trimmed into florets

2 red bell peppers, sliced

1. In a large skillet over medium-high heat, heat the sesame oil.

2. Once the oil is hot, add the onion and cook for about 1 minute. Add the garlic and ginger and cook for another 30 seconds.

3. Add the diced chicken breast and coconut aminos and cook until browned.

4. Add the broccoli and bell pepper to the pan with the chicken and cook until tender.

5. Divide the chicken and veggies between 4 containers.

STORAGE: Once cooled, store in covered containers in the refrigerator for up to 5 days. To reheat, microwave for 2 to 3 minutes.

SMART SHOPPING: Streamline your grocery list and prep by opting for frozen stir-fry veggies in place of fresh vegetables. Thaw the vegetables and then add them in step 4 in place of the broccoli and bell pepper.

Per Serving (1 container): Calories: 309; Fat: 11g; Protein: 31g; Total Carbs: 23g; Fiber: 6g; Sodium: 525mg; Iron: 2g

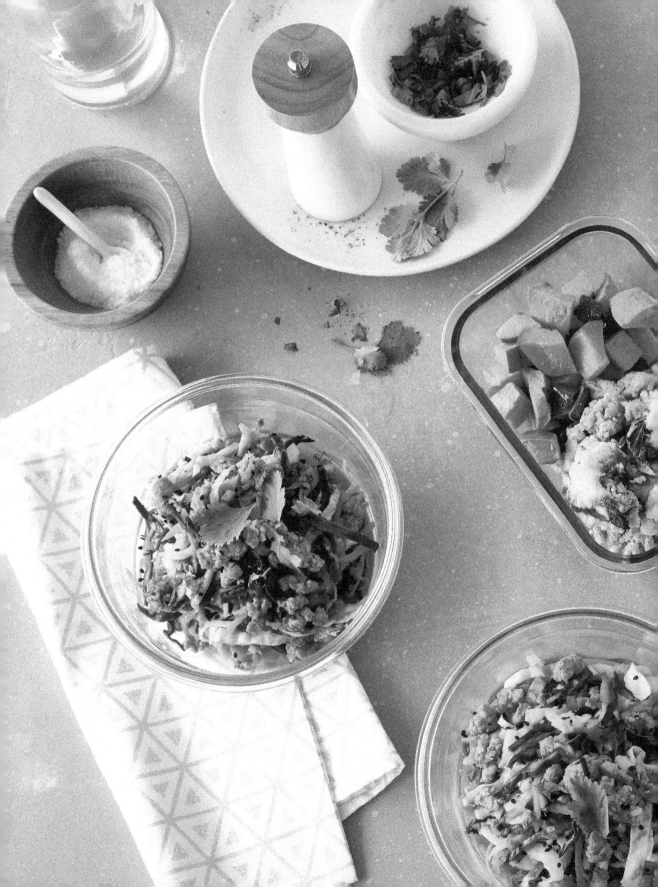

The Athlete

This meal prep plan was designed to support the nutritional needs of active Paleo eaters who regularly work out. With a focus on more carbs and protein, this plan includes breakfast, lunch, and dinner recipes that will keep you energized throughout your workouts.

In order to support high-intensity exercise, it is important to load up on carbohydrates, which can be challenging when you are gluten-free. That is why many of the recipes in this plan include complex carbohydrates like sweet potatoes. It is also important to get enough protein. This performance-based plan is far more enticing than a typical meal prep of grilled chicken and broccoli. In fact, it is packed full of delicious protein-rich recipes like Fish Taco Bowls (page 54), Honey Sesame Chicken with Broccolini (page 52), and Chicken Fajita Bowls (page 61).

If you are looking to pack in even more macronutrients, I recommend prepping high-protein snacks like Beef Jerky (page 144) and Almond Butter Bars (page 136) to consume throughout the week as needed to support your caloric intake needs. And don't forget to drink enough water!

WEEK ONE

	BREAKFAST	LUNCH	DINNER
MONDAY	Egg, Turkey, and Spinach Scramble with Roasted Sweet Potatoes (page 49)	Honey Sesame Chicken with Broccolini (page 52)	Fish Taco Bowls (page 54)
TUESDAY	*Leftover* Egg, Turkey, and Spinach Scramble with Roasted Sweet Potatoes	Cajun Chicken, Broccoli, and Sweet Potatoes (page 47)	*Leftover* Fish Taco Bowls
WEDNESDAY	*Leftover* Egg, Turkey, and Spinach Scramble with Roasted Sweet Potatoes	*Leftover* Honey Sesame Chicken with Broccolini	*Leftover* Cajun Chicken, Broccoli, and Sweet Potatoes
THURSDAY	*Leftover* Egg, Turkey, and Spinach Scramble with Roasted Sweet Potatoes	*Leftover* Cajun Chicken, Broccoli, and Sweet Potatoes	*Leftover* Honey Sesame Chicken with Broccolini
FRIDAY	*Leftover* Egg, Turkey, and Spinach Scramble with Roasted Sweet Potatoes	*Leftover* Honey Sesame Chicken with Broccolini	*Leftover* Cajun Chicken, Broccoli, and Sweet Potatoes

Shopping List

Pantry

- Black pepper
- Cajun seasoning
- Chicken broth (⅓ cup)
- Chili powder
- Coconut aminos
- Garlic powder
- Honey
- Oil, extra-virgin olive
- Oil, sesame
- Paprika
- Sea salt

Produce

- Broccoli (1 head)
- Broccolini (2 heads)
- Cabbage, purple (1 head)
- Cilantro (1 bunch)
- Garlic (1 head)
- Ginger
- Lime (1)
- Mango (1)
- Onion, red (2)
- Radishes (3)
- Spinach, 1 (10-ounce) bag
- Sweet potatoes (4)

Protein

- Boneless skinless chicken breasts (1 pound)
- Chicken thighs (1 pound)
- Eggs (10)
- Ground turkey (8 ounces)
- Halibut fillets (2)

Equipment List

- Baking sheets
- Cast-iron skillet
- Chef's knife
- Cutting board
- Measuring cups and spoons
- Mixing bowls
- Mixing spoon
- Nonstick skillet
- Parchment paper
- Skillet (oven-safe)
- Spatula
- Tongs
- Whisk

Storage Containers

Cajun Chicken, Broccoli, and Sweet Potatoes: 4 (24-ounce) single-compartment meal prep containers

Egg, Turkey, and Spinach Scramble with Roasted Sweet Potatoes: 5 (24-ounce) single-compartment meal prep containers

Honey Sesame Chicken with Broccolini: 4 (24-ounce) single-compartment meal prep containers

Fish Taco Bowls: 2 (24-ounce) single-compartment meal prep containers

Step-by-Step Prep

1. Prepare steps 1 through 4 of the Cajun Chicken, Broccoli, and Sweet Potatoes (page 47), lining three sheets with parchment paper instead of two.

2. Prepare steps 3 and 4 of the Egg, Turkey, and Spinach Scramble with Roasted Sweet Potatoes (page 49) and steps 5 and 6 of the Cajun Chicken, Broccoli and Sweet Potatoes at the same time.

3. While the sweet potatoes are roasting, complete step 7 of the Cajun Chicken, Broccoli, and Sweet Potatoes, then finish steps 5 through 8 of the Egg, Turkey, and Spinach Scramble.

4. When the sweet potatoes are finished cooking, complete step 8 of the Cajun Chicken, Broccoli and Sweet Potatoes and step 9 of the Egg, Turkey, and Spinach Scramble.

5. While the chicken and broccoli cooks, prepare the Honey Sesame Chicken and Broccolini (page 52) in full, pausing to take the chicken and broccoli out of the oven.

6. Finish step 9 of the Cajun Chicken, Broccoli, and Sweet Potatoes.

7. Prepare the Fish Taco Bowls (page 54) in full.

8. Once the food is cool, close and store all containers in the refrigerator.

Cajun Chicken, Broccoli, and Sweet Potatoes

Serves 4 — Prep time: 15 minutes — Cook time: 40 minutes

If you are short on time, I find sheet pan meals are a quick and easy solution to prep a lot of food in a small amount of time. Not only does this recipe use minimal ingredients and equipment, but cleanup is also a breeze. I love the combination of spicy chicken, crisp broccoli, and perfectly roasted sweet potatoes. To me this is an elevated version of the traditional chicken and broccoli enjoyed by so many athletes.

1 pound boneless skinless chicken breasts, cubed

1½ tablespoons Cajun seasoning

3 tablespoons extra-virgin olive oil, divided

Sea salt

Freshly ground black pepper

2 sweet potatoes, cubed

1 red onion, diced

1 head broccoli, trimmed into florets

1. Preheat the oven to 425°F.

2. Line 2 baking sheets with parchment paper.

3. In a large mixing bowl, combine the chicken, Cajun seasoning, and 1 tablespoon of olive oil. Season with salt and pepper. Toss until evenly coated.

4. Store the chicken in the refrigerator while you prep the remaining ingredients.

5. In a large mixing bowl, combine the sweet potatoes, onion, and 1 tablespoon of olive oil. Season with salt and pepper. Toss until evenly coated.

6. Arrange the sweet potatoes and onions in one layer on the lined baking sheet. Bake for 25 minutes, until golden brown, tossing halfway through.

7. Arrange the broccoli florets on the remaining lined baking sheet, drizzle with the remaining olive oil, and season with salt and pepper. Toss to coat evenly. Arrange the chicken on the same baking sheet in a single layer.

CONTINUED

Cajun Chicken, Broccoli, and Sweet Potatoes

CONTINUED

8. Bake for 15 minutes, until chicken is cooked through.

9. Divide the chicken, broccoli, and sweet potatoes between 4 containers.

STORAGE: Once cooled, store in covered containers in the refrigerator for up to 5 days. To reheat, microwave for 2 to 3 minutes.

SIMPLE SWAP: This recipe can be easily switched up week to week with a variety of seasonings and vegetables. Simply swap the Cajun seasoning for the seasoning of your choice. You can also swap the broccoli for cauliflower, and the sweet potato for butternut squash or another root vegetable.

Per Serving (1 container): Calories: 340; Fat: 14g; Protein: 31g; Total Carbs: 26g; Fiber: 6g; Sodium: 420mg; Iron: 2g

Egg, Turkey, and Spinach Scramble with Roasted Sweet Potatoes

Serves 5 — Prep time: 10 minutes — Cook time: 35 minutes

This recipe is the perfect way to start the day. Packed with two sources of protein, greens, and hearty root vegetables, this breakfast is sure to keep you fueled throughout your day—and your workout. By meal prepping this dish over the weekend you are setting yourself up for success. You can enjoy this scramble in the morning before a workout, or grab it from the refrigerator on the way to the office.

2 sweet potatoes, cubed

1 red onion, diced

2 garlic cloves, minced, divided

2 tablespoons extra-virgin olive oil, divided

1 teaspoon sea salt, divided

½ teaspoon freshly ground black pepper, divided

10 eggs

8 ounces ground turkey

4 cups baby spinach

1. Preheat the oven to 425°F.

2. Line a baking sheet with parchment paper.

3. In a large mixing bowl, combine the sweet potatoes, onion, half of the garlic, and 1 tablespoon of olive oil. Season with ½ teaspoon of salt and ¼ teaspoon of pepper. Toss until evenly coated.

4. Arrange the sweet potatoes and onions in one layer on the lined baking sheet. Bake for 25 minutes, until golden brown, tossing halfway through.

5. In a nonstick skillet, heat the remaining olive oil over medium-high heat. Meanwhile, in a large mixing bowl, whisk together the eggs and remaining salt and pepper. Set aside.

6. Add the ground turkey to the skillet and cook for 3 to 5 minutes. Add the remaining garlic and cook for another minute.

CONTINUED

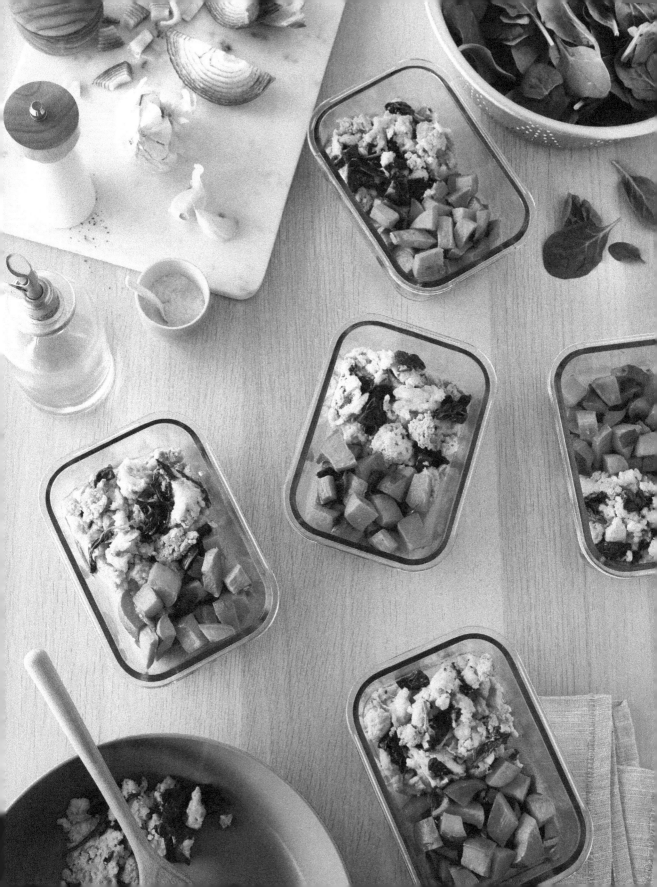

Egg, Turkey, and Spinach Scramble with Roasted Sweet Potatoes

CONTINUED

7. Add the spinach to the skillet and cook for 2 to 3 minutes, until wilted.

8. Add the eggs to the skillet and allow to cook, without stirring, until the mixture begins to set around the edges. Using a spatula, gently stir the eggs, and continue cooking until the egg whites are just cooked through.

9. Divide the scrambled eggs and turkey mixture and sweet potatoes between 5 containers.

STORAGE: Once cooled, store in covered containers in the refrigerator for up to 5 days. To reheat, microwave for 1 to 2 minutes.

SIMPLE SWAP: Switch up this scramble by swapping out the ground turkey for ham. You can also swap the spinach for another veggie of your choice.

Per Serving (1 container): Calories: 342; Fat: 20g; Protein: 25g; Total Carbs: 15g; Fiber: g; Sodium: 670mg; Iron: 3g

Honey Sesame Chicken with Broccolini

Serves 4 — Prep time: 10 minutes — Cook time: 30 minutes

This homemade version of a Chinese takeout favorite gets a makeover. This version is made with chicken thighs baked in a homemade sauce so that it is crisp-tender and packed with tons of flavor. Plus, I swapped out the traditional broccoli florets for broccolini, which reheats beautifully. Looking to beef up this dish to make it a bit heartier? Prep a batch of Cauliflower Rice (page 95).

1 pound chicken thighs, skin-on

Sea salt

Freshly ground black pepper

1 tablespoon extra-virgin olive oil

⅓ cup chicken broth

3 tablespoons coconut aminos

3 tablespoons honey

2 tablespoons sesame oil, divided

1 tablespoon grated fresh ginger

2 garlic cloves, minced

2 bunches broccolini, ends trimmed

1. Preheat the oven to 425°F.

2. Season the chicken with salt and pepper.

3. In a large oven-safe skillet, heat the olive oil over medium-high heat. Add the chicken to the skillet, skin-side down, and cook for 5 minutes until golden brown.

4. Meanwhile, in a large mixing bowl, whisk together the chicken broth, coconut aminos, honey, 1 tablespoon of sesame oil, ginger, and garlic.

5. Flip the chicken and add the broth mixture to the skillet. Bring to a simmer.

6. Transfer the skillet to the oven and cook for 15 minutes, or until the chicken is cooked through and reaches an internal temperature of 165°F.

7. Meanwhile, in a large mixing bowl, toss the broccolini in the remaining sesame oil. Season with salt and pepper.

8. Arrange the broccolini in one layer on a baking sheet. Bake for 10 minutes, tossing halfway through.

9. Divide the chicken and broccolini between 4 containers.

STORAGE: Once cooled, store in covered containers in the refrigerator for up to 5 days. To reheat, microwave for 2 to 3 minutes.

COOKING HACK: Speed up the cooking time for this dish by using diced chicken breast or chicken thighs in place of the full chicken thighs in this recipe.

Per Serving (1 container): Calories: 582; Fat: 35g; Protein: 39g; Total Carbs: 28g; Fiber: 5g; Sodium: 1075mg; Iron: 2g

Fish Taco Bowls

Serves 2 — Prep time: 10 minutes — Cook time: 10 minutes

This is not your typical meal prep recipe. In fact, I find that many people steer away from fish when meal prepping for fear that it will not reheat well. I meal prep fish in small portions so that it is enjoyed within 3 days. I also recommend fish for dinner so that you can reheat the fish at home in the oven versus in the office microwave. Bulk up this bowl and make it even more calorie dense by serving it with Cauliflower Rice (page 95) and fresh avocado, if desired.

½ teaspoon chili powder

½ teaspoon paprika

½ teaspoon sea salt

⅛ teaspoon freshly ground black pepper

⅛ teaspoon garlic powder

2 halibut fillets

1 tablespoon extra-virgin olive oil

½ head purple cabbage, shredded

3 radishes, sliced

½ mango, cubed

1 tablespoon finely chopped cilantro

1 lime, halved

1. In a small mixing bowl, add the chili powder, paprika, salt, pepper, and garlic powder. Mix well. Rub the fish with the spice mixture.

2. In a large cast iron skillet, heat the olive oil over medium-high heat.

3. Cook the fish in the skillet for 5 minutes. Flip fish and cook for another 5 minutes, until cooked through. Slice if desired.

4. Divide the cabbage, radishes, mango, cilantro, and lime between 2 containers. Top with the fish.

STORAGE: Once cooled, store in covered containers in the refrigerator for up to 3 days. To reheat, remove the fish from the container and microwave for 2 to 3 minutes or bake in a 400°F oven for 8 to 10 minutes.

SIMPLE SWAP: If halibut is not available at your local market, tilapia, flounder, and cod all work well in this recipe. You can also swap out the fish for another protein of your choice. Chicken works great!

Per Serving (1 container): Calories: 255; Fat: 8g; Protein: 20g; Total Carbs: 30g; Fiber: 8g; Sodium: 699mg; Iron: 2g

	BREAKFAST	LUNCH	DINNER
MONDAY	Spicy Sausage Patties and Veggies (page 58)	Chicken Fajita Bowls (page 61)	Sheet Pan Greek Chicken and Vegetables (page 60)
TUESDAY	*Leftover* Spicy Sausage Patties and Veggies	Pork Egg Roll Bowls (page 63)	*Leftover* Sheet Pan Greek Chicken and Vegetables
WEDNESDAY	*Leftover* Spicy Sausage Patties and Veggies	*Leftover* Chicken Fajita Bowls	*Leftover* Pork Egg Roll Bowls
THURSDAY	*Leftover* Spicy Sausage Patties and Veggies	*Leftover* Chicken Fajita Bowls	*Leftover* Sheet Pan Greek Chicken and Vegetables
FRIDAY	*Leftover* Spicy Sausage Patties and Veggies	*Leftover* Sheet Pan Greek Chicken and Vegetables	*Leftover* Chicken Fajita Bowls

Shopping List

Pantry

- ☐ Allspice
- ☐ Black pepper
- ☐ Cayenne pepper
- ☐ Chili powder
- ☐ Coconut aminos
- ☐ Cumin
- ☐ Fennel seeds, crushed
- ☐ Greek seasoning
- ☐ Oil, extra-virgin olive
- ☐ Oil, sesame
- ☐ Paprika
- ☐ Sea salt
- ☐ Sesame seeds
- ☐ Vinegar, rice

Produce

- Brussels sprouts (1 pound)
- Cabbage, green (1 head)
- Cabbage, red (1 head)
- Carrot (1)
- Cauliflower (1 head)
- Cilantro (1 bunch)
- Cucumber (1)
- Dill
- Garlic (1 head)
- Ginger
- Lemon (2)
- Onion, red (3)
- Onion, white (1)
- Pepper, green bell (1)
- Pepper, red bell (3)
- Pepper, yellow bell (1)
- Sweet potato (1)
- Zucchini (1)

Protein

- Boneless chicken breast (2 pounds)
- Coconut milk yogurt, plain, unsweetened (1 cup)
- Ground pork (1½ pounds)

Equipment List

- Baking sheets
- Chef's knife
- Cutting board
- Food processor
- Measuring cups and spoons
- Mixing bowls
- Mixing spoon
- Parchment paper
- Skillet
- Spatula
- Tongs

Storage Containers

Spicy Sausage Patties and Veggies: 5 (24-ounce) single-compartment meal prep containers

Sheet Pan Greek Chicken and Vegetables: 4 (24-ounce) single-compartment meal prep containers and 4 (2-ounce) sauce cups

Chicken Fajita Bowls: 4 (24-ounce) single-compartment meal prep containers

Pork Egg Roll Bowls: 2 (24-ounce) single-compartment meal prep containers

Step-by-Step Prep

1. Prepare the Spicy Sausage Patties and Veggies (page 58) in full.

2. Prepare the Sheet Pan Greek Chicken and Vegetables (page 60) through step 5.

3. While the chicken and vegetables are roasting, prepare the Chicken Fajita Bowls (page 61) in full, pausing to remove the chicken and vegetables from the oven when done.

4. Complete step 6 of the Sheet Pan Greek Chicken and Vegetables.

5. Prepare the Pork Egg Roll Bowls (page 63) in full.

6. Once the food is cool, close and store the containers in the refrigerator.

Spicy Sausage Patties and Veggies

Serves 5 — Prep time: 15 minutes — Cook time: 25 minutes

Homemade sausage patties sound intimidating, but the truth is they are as simple to assemble as meatballs. Simply season your choice of protein, and then sear them in a skillet to maximize flavor. This spicy sausage recipe uses ground pork, but you can easily swap it for ground beef or chicken if you prefer.

1 sweet potato, peeled and cubed

1½ red onions, diced, divided

1 pound Brussels sprouts, trimmed and halved lengthwise

4 tablespoons extra-virgin olive oil, divided

Sea salt

Freshly ground black pepper

1 pound ground pork

½ teaspoon crushed fennel seeds

¼ teaspoon cumin

⅛ teaspoon allspice

Pinch red cayenne pepper

1. Preheat the oven to 425°F.
2. Line a baking sheet with parchment paper.
3. In a large mixing bowl, combine the sweet potato, 1 onion, Brussels sprouts, and 2 tablespoons of olive oil. Season with salt and pepper. Toss until evenly coated.
4. Arrange the vegetables in one layer on the lined baking sheet. Bake for 20 to 25 minutes, until golden brown, tossing halfway through.
5. In a large skillet, heat 1 tablespoon of olive oil over medium heat. Add half of the remaining onion and cook for 2 minutes, until soft and translucent. Remove from the heat.
6. In a large mixing bowl, combine the ground pork, remaining onion, fennel seeds, cumin, allspice, and cayenne pepper. Season with salt and pepper and mix well. Form mixture into 10 patties.
7. In a large skillet, heat the remaining olive oil over medium heat. Put half of the sausage patties in the pan and cook 2 to 3 minutes per side. Repeat with remaining sausage patties.

8. Divide the sausage patties, Brussels sprouts, and sweet potatoes between 5 containers.

STORAGE: Once cooled, store in covered containers in the refrigerator for up to 5 days. To reheat, microwave for 2 to 3 minutes.

SIMPLE SWAP: If you are short on time and don't want to make sausage patties from scratch, use bacon instead, or skip the sausage patties and enjoy the veggies with a side of scrambled eggs.

Per Serving (1 container): Calories: 282; Fat: 15g; Protein: 23g; Total Carbs: 17g; Fiber: 5g; Sodium: 129mg; Iron: 2g

Sheet Pan Greek Chicken and Vegetables

Serves 4 — Prep time: 30 minutes — Cook time: 25 minutes

The secret to sheet pan meals is they all follow the same formula—protein, veggies, seasoning, and a sprinkle of oil to ensure it all crisps up. No need to keep things neat here; simply toss the ingredients together and let the oven do the work for you.

1 cup Tzatziki (page 90)

1 pound chicken breasts, diced

1 red bell pepper, diced

1 yellow bell pepper, diced

1 zucchini, thickly sliced

1 red onion, thickly sliced

2 tablespoons extra-virgin olive oil

2 tablespoons freshly squeezed lemon juice

4 garlic cloves, minced

2 tablespoons Greek seasoning

1 teaspoon sea salt

1. Prepare the tzatziki and set aside.
2. Preheat the oven to 425°F.
3. Line a baking sheet with parchment paper.
4. In a large mixing bowl, combine all of the ingredients except the tzatziki and toss until evenly coated.
5. Arrange the chicken and vegetables in one layer on the lined baking sheet. Bake for 20 to 25 minutes, until golden brown, tossing halfway through with tongs.
6. Divide the chicken and veggies between 4 containers. Divide the tzatziki into 4 (2-ounce) cups with lids.

STORAGE: Once cooled, store in covered containers in the refrigerator for up to 5 days. To reheat, microwave for 2 to 3 minutes. Top with the tzatziki before enjoying.

COOKING HACK: Serve this dish with tabbouleh by taking the Cauliflower Rice (page 95) and adding ½ of a cucumber (diced), 1 tomato (diced), 1 cup of chopped parsley, and 2 tablespoons of freshly squeezed lemon juice to the cooked cauliflower. Toss until well combined.

Per Serving (1 container): Calories: 284; Fat: 14g; Protein: 28g; Total Carbs: 16g; Fiber: 3g; Sodium: 909mg; Iron: 1g

Chicken Fajita Bowls

Serves 4 — Prep time: 45 minutes — Cook time: 10 minutes

Fajitas are often served deconstructed, and you assemble them as you eat. If you want to keep with tradition, you can prep your containers so that the chicken, peppers, and rice are all arranged in neat rows. However, I love letting all of the flavors meld together so that there is a little bit of everything in each bite! Just like any stir-fry, you can swap out the sauce, protein, and veggies in this recipe to create something new so you have endless meal prep possibilities.

Cauliflower Rice (page 95)

1 tablespoon extra-virgin olive oil

1 pound boneless chicken breast, sliced

2 red bell peppers, cored, seeded, and thinly sliced

1 green bell pepper, cored, seeded, and thinly sliced

1 onion, thinly sliced

1 teaspoon paprika

½ teaspoon chili powder

¼ teaspoon cumin

Sea salt

Freshly ground black pepper

1. Prepare the cauliflower rice and set aside.
2. In a large skillet over medium heat, heat the oil.
3. When the oil is hot, add the chicken, bell peppers, and onion. Sauté for 30 seconds.
4. Add the paprika, chili powder, and cumin to the pan, and season with salt and pepper. Stir to combine all of the ingredients.
5. Sauté the mixture until the chicken is fully cooked through, about 8 minutes, stirring regularly.
6. Divide the chicken mixture and cauliflower rice evenly between 4 containers.

STORAGE: Once cooled, store in covered containers in the refrigerator for up to 5 days. To reheat, microwave for 2 to 3 minutes.

SIMPLE SWAP: Switch things up and enjoy these Chicken Fajitas rolled up in iceberg or romaine lettuce. Or bulk up this bowl and make it even more calorie dense by serving with Cauliflower Rice (page 95).

Per Serving (1 container): Calories: 269; Fat: 11g; Protein: 30g; Total Carbs: 16g; Fiber: 6g; Sodium: 187mg; Iron: 2g

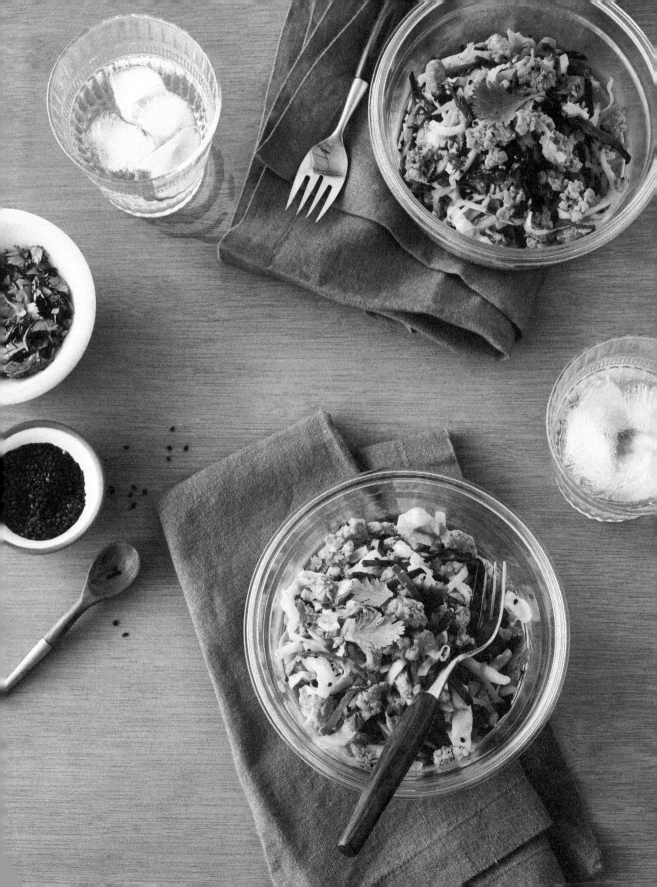

Pork Egg Roll Bowls

Serves 2 — Prep time: 10 minutes — Cook time: 15 minutes

From burrito and taco bowls, to noodle and Buddha bowls, these days all of my favorite dishes have been transformed into a trendy bowl. So, it was a no-brainier to deconstruct an egg roll into a bowl. With this combination of crunchy cabbage, flavorful pork, and bold spices, you won't even miss a deep-fried egg roll wrapper. Just like the best Chinese takeout, you can enjoy this dish hot or cold.

½ tablespoon sesame oil

2 garlic cloves, minced

1 tablespoon minced ginger

8 ounces ground pork

1 carrot, peeled and shredded

1 cup shredded red cabbage

1 cup shredded green cabbage

1 tablespoon coconut aminos

½ tablespoon rice wine vinegar

2 tablespoons minced cilantro

Sesame seeds, to taste

1. In a large skillet, heat the sesame oil over medium heat. Add the garlic and ginger and cook for about 30 seconds, until fragrant.
2. Add the pork and cook for 6 to 8 minutes, until cooked through.
3. Add the carrot, red cabbage, green cabbage, coconut aminos, and rice vinegar. Cook for another 3 to 5 minutes, stirring frequently.
4. Divide the mixture between 2 containers. Top with cilantro and sesame seeds.

STORAGE: Once cooled, store in covered containers in the refrigerator for up to 5 days. To reheat, microwave for 2 to 3 minutes. You can also enjoy this dish cold, without reheating, if you prefer.

SMART SHOPPING: These days, you can find most vegetables diced and shredded to cut down on prep work. While I don't recommend purchased pre-prepped vegetables regularly, I find that it doesn't impact the flavor or freshness of the carrot and cabbage in this dish.

Per Serving (1 container): Calories: 257; Fat: 11g; Protein: 27g; Total Carbs: 14g; Fiber: 4g; Sodium: 330mg; Iron: 2g

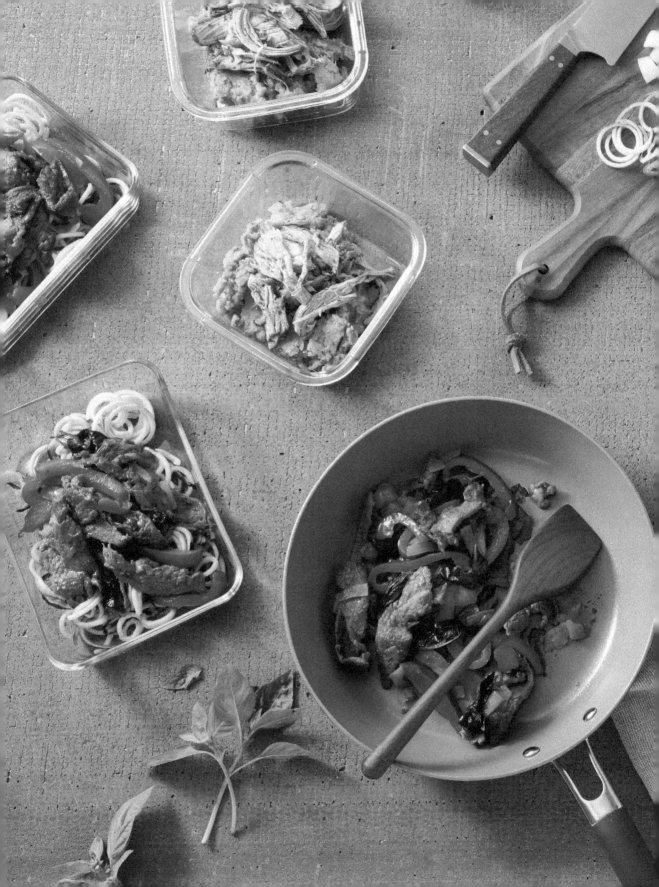

Paleo as a Lifestyle

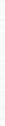

This meal prep plan is geared toward those who are not new to Paleo but want to make it as easy (and enticing) as possible to continue to follow the Paleo diet. I basically designed this plan from all of my personal favorites!

This prep will offer breakfast, lunch, and dinner options so that you can continue to enjoy the benefits of the Paleo diet without getting bored. With recipes like Chicken Curry and Cauliflower Rice (page 73), Chicken and Veggie Fried Cauliflower Rice (page 82), and Thai Basil Beef and Noodles (page 83), this plan is full of takeout-inspired favorites that are packed with flavor. The recipes throughout this plan are creative and fun, perfect if you are bored with traditional Paleo recipes and want to add some creativity and ingenuity into your kitchen.

WEEK ONE

	BREAKFAST	LUNCH	DINNER
MONDAY	Turkey, Sweet Potato, and Kale Hash (page 71)	Teriyaki Turkey Meatballs and Cauliflower Rice (page 69)	Chicken Curry and Cauliflower Rice (page 73)
TUESDAY	Leftover Turkey, Sweet Potato, and Kale Hash	Leftover Teriyaki Turkey Meatballs and Cauliflower Rice	Jamaican Jerk Chicken and Mashed Plantains (page 75)
WEDNESDAY	Leftover Turkey, Sweet Potato, and Kale Hash	Leftover Chicken Curry and Cauliflower Rice	Leftover Teriyaki Turkey Meatballs and Cauliflower Rice
THURSDAY	Leftover Turkey, Sweet Potato, and Kale Hash	Leftover Jamaican Jerk Chicken and Mashed Plantains	Leftover Chicken Curry and Cauliflower Rice
FRIDAY	Leftover Turkey, Sweet Potato, and Kale Hash	Leftover Chicken Curry and Cauliflower Rice	Leftover Jamaican Jerk Chicken and Mashed Plantains

Shopping List

Pantry

- Allspice
- Black pepper
- Chicken broth
- Cinnamon
- Flour, arrowroot
- Flour, coconut
- Coconut milk, full fat (2 cans)
- Garlic powder
- Ground ginger
- Ground sage
- Honey
- Nutmeg
- Oil, coconut
- Oil, extra-virgin olive
- Onion powder
- Orange juice
- Paprika
- Sea salt
- Tomato paste
- Turmeric
- Thyme

Produce

- Cauliflower (2 heads)
- Garlic (1 head)
- Kale (1 bunch)
- Lime (1)
- Onion, white (1)
- Pepper, green bell (2)
- Plantains, brown (3)
- Sweet potatoes (2)

Protein

- Boneless skinless chicken breast (2 pounds)
- Ground turkey (2 pounds)

Equipment List

- Baking sheets
- Chef's knife
- Cutting board
- Food processor
- Measuring cups and spoons
- Mixing bowls
- Mixing spoon
- Parchment paper
- Pressure cooker or slow cooker
- Saucepan
- Skillet (with lid)
- Spatula
- Tongs
- Whisk

Storage Containers

Teriyaki Turkey Meatballs and Cauliflower Rice: 3 (24-ounce) single-compartment meal prep containers

Turkey, Sweet Potato, and Kale Hash: 5 (24-ounce) single-compartment meal prep containers

Chicken Curry and Cauliflower Rice: 4 (24-ounce) single-compartment meal prep containers

Jamaican Jerk Chicken and Mashed Plantains: 3 (24-ounce) single-compartment meal prep containers

Step-by-Step Prep

1. Prepare the Turkey Teriyaki Meatballs (page 69) in full, making a double batch of the Cauliflower Rice (page 95).

2. Prepare the Turkey, Sweet Potato, and Kale Hash (page 71) in full.

3. Prepare the Chicken Curry and Cauliflower Rice (page 73) in full, omitting step 3.

4. While the chicken curry is cooking, prepare steps 3 through 5 of Jamaican Jerk Chicken and Mashed Plantains (page 75).

5. When the chicken curry is finished cooking, prepare steps 1 and 2 of the Jamaican Jerk Chicken, then finish steps 6 and 7.

6. Once the food is cool, close and store the containers in the refrigerator.

Teriyaki Turkey Meatballs and Cauliflower Rice

Serves 3 — Prep time: 40 minutes — Cook time: 25 minutes

In this recipe, juicy meatballs are smothered in a thick, sticky, and sweet teriyaki sauce and served with a side of cauliflower rice. Once you get the hang of this super easy, homemade teriyaki sauce, not only can you use it as a sauce for a variety of beef, pork, and chicken meatballs, but you can also use it with chicken breast, salmon, and more!

1 pound ground turkey

1½ teaspoons garlic powder, divided

1¼ teaspoons ground ginger, divided

1 teaspoon sea salt

½ teaspoon freshly ground black pepper

2 teaspoons coconut flour

1 tablespoon coconut oil

½ cup coconut aminos

2 teaspoons honey

2 tablespoons orange juice

1 teaspoon arrowroot flour

Cauliflower Rice (page 95)

1. Preheat the oven to 400°F.
2. Line a baking sheet with parchment paper.
3. In a large mixing bowl, combine the ground turkey, 1 teaspoon of garlic powder, 1 teaspoon of ground ginger, 1 teaspoon of salt, ½ teaspoon of pepper, coconut flour, and coconut oil. Mix well and roll into 12 meatballs.
4. Arrange the meatballs in one layer on the lined baking sheet. Bake for 20 to 25 minutes, until golden brown, flipping meatballs halfway through.
5. Meanwhile, in a small saucepan over medium heat, combine the coconut aminos, honey, and orange juice for 3 minutes. Whisk in the arrowroot flour, reduce heat to low, and simmer for 3 minutes until the sauce thickens.
6. Prepare the cauliflower rice and set aside.
7. Remove the meatballs from the oven and toss in the sauce until evenly coated.
8. Divide the cauliflower rice and meatballs between 3 containers.

CONTINUED

Teriyaki Turkey Meatballs and Cauliflower Rice

CONTINUED

STORAGE: Once cooled, store in covered containers in the refrigerator for up to 5 days. To reheat, microwave for 2 to 3 minutes.

SMART SHOPPING: Arrowroot flour is a starch extracted from tropical plants and is a common Paleo alternative to corn starch. It is typically found in the baking aisle near the gluten-free flours. Bob's Red Mill is a brand that I like to use.

Per Serving (1 container): Calories: 571; Fat: 27g; Protein: 46g; Total Carbs: 35g; Fiber: 5g; Sodium: 2158mg; Iron: 4g

Turkey, Sweet Potato, and Kale Hash

Serves 5 — Prep time: 10 minutes — Cook time: 25 minutes

Breakfast used to be my least favorite meal of the day because I was stuck in an egg rut. When I first started eating Paleo, it was difficult to think outside of the box for a hearty meal that didn't center around eggs. As I have grown in my Paleo journey, I have found ways to introduce protein into breakfast through other ingredients. In this dish, turkey, sweet potatoes, and kale are brought together with a warm, comforting spice blend.

**1 teaspoon
ground cinnamon**

**½ teaspoon
onion powder**

**½ teaspoon
garlic powder**

½ teaspoon ground sage

½ teaspoon turmeric

**2 tablespoons
extra-virgin olive
oil, divided**

1 pound ground turkey

Sea salt

**Freshly ground
black pepper**

**2 sweet potatoes, peeled
and diced**

3 cups chopped kale

1 tablespoon water

1. In a small bowl, combine the cinnamon, onion powder, garlic powder, ground sage, and turmeric. Stir to combine all of the ingredients.

2. In a large skillet, heat 1 tablespoon of olive oil over medium-high heat. Add the ground turkey and season with salt, pepper, and half of the spice mixture. Cook for 5 to 8 minutes, until browned.

3. Transfer the turkey to a plate. Heat the remaining olive oil over medium-high heat. Add the sweet potatoes and season with salt, pepper, and the remaining spice mixture. Cook for 5 minutes, stirring frequently.

4. Lower the heat to medium and cover the skillet. Cook for another 5 to 8 minutes, until the potatoes are soft.

5. Uncover and add the kale, water, and turkey. Cover the skillet for 2 minutes. Uncover and cook for another 2 minutes, stirring frequently.

6. Divide the hash evenly between 5 containers.

CONTINUED

Turkey, Sweet Potato, and Kale Hash

CONTINUED

STORAGE: Once cooled, store in covered containers in the refrigerator for up to 5 days. To reheat, microwave for 2 to 3 minutes.

COOKING HACK: To make this recipe even easier and faster, I recommend partially cooking the diced sweet potato in the microwave. To partially cook vegetables in the microwave, place chopped veggies in a microwave-safe bowl and loosely cover. Microwave on high for 5 to 7 minutes.

Per Serving (1 container): Calories: 295; Fat: 16g; Protein: 26g; Total Carbs: 12g; Fiber: 3g; Sodium: 149mg; Iron: 2g

Chicken Curry and Cauliflower Rice

Serves 4 — Prep time: 35 minutes — Cook time: 25 minutes

This curry is rich and warming, with a little spice and a whole lot of coconut. One of my favorite meal prep hacks is using a pressure cooker to make quick work of proteins, soups, and stews. In this recipe, the pressure cooker brings together simple ingredients to create a bold stew bursting with flavor.

1 pound boneless, skinless chicken breast

1 cup chicken broth

2 garlic cloves, minced

½ onion, diced

2 green bell peppers, diced

1 tablespoon tomato paste

1½ tablespoons curry powder

1 teaspoon ground turmeric

½ teaspoon sea salt

Cauliflower Rice (page 95)

1 (15-ounce) can full-fat coconut milk

1. Add the chicken, chicken broth, garlic, onion, peppers, tomato paste, curry powder, ground turmeric, and salt to a pressure cooker pot.

2. Cook on high pressure for 8 minutes, then let the pressure release naturally for 10 minutes.

3. While the curry is cooking, prepare the cauliflower rice and set aside.

4. Carefully remove the pressure lid and shred the chicken with 2 forks.

5. Add the coconut milk and set the sauté setting on the pressure cooker to low. Let the chicken simmer for 5 minutes.

6. Divide the cauliflower rice and chicken mixture between 4 containers.

STORAGE: Once cooled, store in covered containers in the refrigerator for up to 5 days. To reheat, microwave for 2 to 3 minutes.

COOKING HACK: If you do not have a pressure cooker, you can make this recipe in a slow cooker. Cook the chicken on high for 3 to 4 hours, or low for 6 to 8 hours.

Per Serving (1 container): Calories: 412; Fat: 23g; Protein: 32g; Total Carbs: 18g; Fiber: 6g; Sodium: 702mg; Iron: 3g

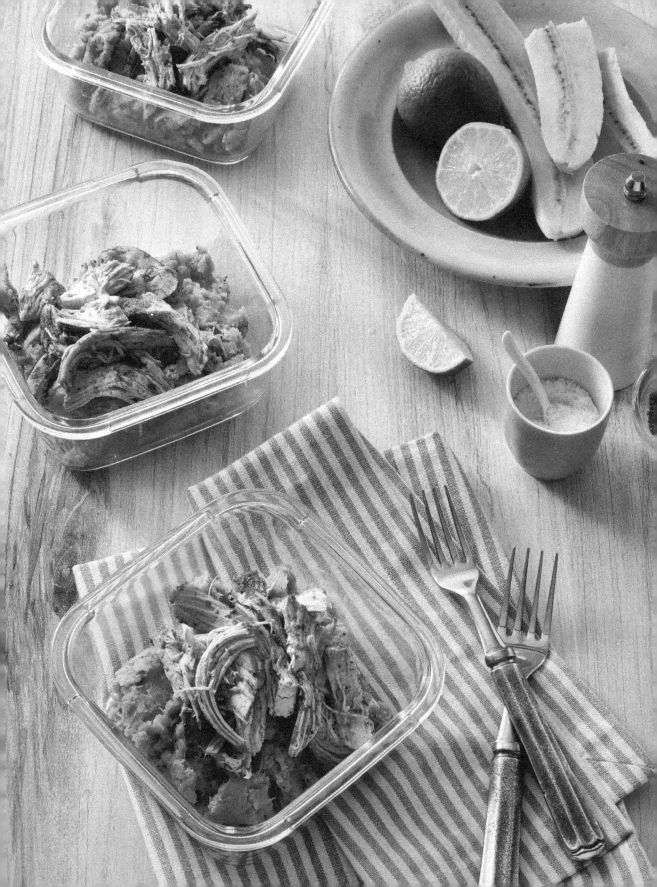

Jamaican Jerk Chicken and Mashed Plantains

Serves 3 — Prep time: 10 minutes — Cook time: 25 minutes

This recipe is the perfect blend of flavor and texture. While you're building flavor by pressure cooking your chicken and spices, you are also pulling together a soft plantain mash with a few simple ingredients.

1 pound boneless, skinless chicken breast

1 cup chicken broth

2 tablespoons freshly squeezed lime juice

1 teaspoon allspice

1 teaspoon nutmeg

1 teaspoon garlic powder

1 teaspoon thyme

1 teaspoon paprika

2 tablespoons coconut oil

3 brown plantains, peeled, sliced in half lengthwise

½ teaspoon cinnamon

½ teaspoon sea salt

4 tablespoons full-fat canned coconut milk

1. Put the chicken, chicken broth, lime juice, allspice, nutmeg, garlic powder, thyme, and paprika in a pressure cooker pot.

2. Cook on high pressure for 10 minutes, then let the pressure release naturally for 10 minutes.

3. Meanwhile, in a large skillet heat the coconut oil over medium-high heat.

4. Add the plantains and sprinkle with the cinnamon and salt. Cook for 5 minutes, flip, and cook for another 5 minutes, or until soft.

5. Remove the plantains from the stove and use a food processor or blender to puree the plantains and coconut milk.

6. When the chicken is done cooking, carefully remove the pressure lid and shred the chicken.

7. Divide the plantains and chicken between 3 containers.

STORAGE: Once cooled, store in covered containers in the refrigerator for up to 5 days. To reheat, microwave for 2 to 3 minutes.

COOKING HACK: You can make this recipe in a slow cooker. Cook the chicken on high for 3 to 4 hours, or on low for 6 to 8 hours.

Per Serving (1 container): Calories: 642; Fat: 17g; Protein: 39g; Total Carbs: 90g; Fiber: 6g; Sodium: 788mg; Iron: 3g

	BREAKFAST	LUNCH	DINNER
MONDAY	Breakfast Tacos (page 79)	Chicken and Veggie Fried Cauliflower Rice (page 82)	Crispy Baked Fish and Parsnip Chips (page 80)
TUESDAY	*Leftover* Breakfast Tacos	Thai Basil Beef and Noodles (page 83)	*Leftover* Crispy Baked Fish and Parsnip Chips
WEDNESDAY	*Leftover* Breakfast Tacos	*Leftover* Chicken and Veggie Fried Cauliflower Rice	*Leftover* Thai Basil Beef and Noodles
THURSDAY	*Leftover* Breakfast Tacos	*Leftover* Thai Basil Beef and Noodles	*Leftover* Chicken and Veggie Fried Cauliflower Rice
FRIDAY	*Leftover* Breakfast Tacos	*Leftover* Chicken and Veggie Fried Cauliflower Rice	*Leftover* Thai Basil Beef and Noodles

Shopping List

Pantry

- ☐ Basil, dried
- ☐ Black pepper
- ☐ Cayenne pepper
- ☐ Chili powder
- ☐ Coconut aminos
- ☐ Cumin
- ☐ Fish sauce
- ☐ Flour, arrowroot
- ☐ Flour, coconut
- ☐ Garlic powder
- ☐ Oil, avocado
- ☐ Oil, coconut
- ☐ Oil, extra-virgin olive
- ☐ Onion powder
- ☐ Paprika
- ☐ Sea salt

Produce

- Basil leaves (1 cup)
- Carrot (1)
- Cauliflower (1 head)
- Cilantro (1 bunch)
- Garlic (1 head)
- Lemon (1)
- Lime (1)
- Onion, red (2)
- Onion, white (1)
- Parsnip (1)
- Peas (½ cup)
- Pepper, green bell (1)
- Pepper, red bell (2)
- Sweet potatoes (2)
- Thai chiles (2)
- Zucchini (2)

Protein

- Boneless chicken breast (1 pound)
- Cod (2 pounds)
- Eggs (8)
- Flank steak (2 pounds)

Equipment List

- Aluminum foil
- Baking sheets
- Chef's knife
- Cutting board
- Food processor
- Measuring cups and spoons
- Mixing bowls
- Mixing spoon
- Nonstick skillet (large and small)
- Parchment paper
- Spatula
- Spiralizer
- Tongs

Storage Containers

Breakfast Tacos: 5 (24-ounce) single-compartment meal prep containers

Crispy Baked Fish and Parsnip Chips: 2 (24-ounce) single-compartment meal prep containers

Chicken and Veggie Fried Cauliflower Rice: 4 (24-ounce) single-compartment meal prep containers

Thai Basil Beef and Noodles: 4 (24-ounce) single-compartment meal prep containers

Step-by-Step Prep

1. Prepare the Breakfast Tacos (page 79) in full.

2. Increase oven temperature to 450°F and prepare the Crispy Baked Fish and Parsnip Chips (page 80) through step 7.

3. While the fish is baking, prepare the Cauliflower Rice (page 95) in full.

4. Complete step 8 of the Crispy Baked Fish and Parsnip Chips, then continue preparing steps 2 through 7 of the Chicken and Veggie Fried Cauliflower Rice (page 82).

5. Prepare the Thai Basil Beef and Noodles (page 83) in full.

6. Once the food is cool, close and store the containers in the refrigerator.

Breakfast Tacos

Serves 5 — Prep time: 30 minutes — Cook time: 35 minutes

These breakfast tacos turn the traditional breakfast taco inside out, literally. Here I use Egg Wraps (page 97) as the shell for the taco and fill them full of hearty veggies. Like many of my recipes, you can easily customize this dish by swapping the veggies. You can also top with hot sauce, avocado, or even coconut milk yogurt to pack in more flavor.

2 sweet potatoes, peeled and diced

1 green bell pepper, diced

1 red onion, diced

1 teaspoon chili powder

1 teaspoon cumin

½ teaspoon garlic powder

1 tablespoon extra-virgin olive oil

Sea salt

Freshly ground black pepper

5 Egg Wraps (page 97)

Cilantro, for garnish

1 lime, cut into wedges

1. Preheat the oven to 425°F.
2. Line a baking sheet with parchment paper.
3. In a large mixing bowl, combine the sweet potatoes, bell pepper, onion, chili powder, cumin, garlic powder, and olive oil. Season with salt and pepper. Toss until evenly coated.
4. Arrange the vegetables in one layer on the lined baking sheet. Bake for 25 minutes, until golden brown, tossing halfway through.
5. Prepare the egg wraps and set aside.
6. Place an egg wrap in the bottom of each of the 5 containers. Divide the roasted vegetables evenly to fill each egg wrap. Top with cilantro and a lime wedge.

STORAGE: Once cooled, store in covered containers in the refrigerator for up to 5 days. To reheat, microwave for 2 to 3 minutes.

SIMPLE SWAP: If you don't have egg wraps already made or you are looking for a breakfast option without eggs, simply omit the wraps and enjoy the hash.

Per Serving (1 container): Calories: 183; Fat: 10g; Protein: 7g; Total Carbs: 16g; Fiber: 3g; Sodium: 132mg; Iron: 1g

Crispy Baked Fish
and Parsnip Chips

Serves 2 — Prep time: 15 minutes — Cook time: 30 minutes

A twist on a classic, this baked fish recipe was inspired by the fried favorite. Flaky fish with a crisp breading pairs perfectly with baked parsnip chips. While this recipe can be reheated in the microwave, I like to use the toaster oven because it heats up quickly and preserves the texture of the dish. Serve the fish and chips on their own or on top of a bed of arugula.

1 large parsnip, peeled and cut into thick fries

1 tablespoon avocado oil

⅓ cup coconut flour

¾ cup almond flour

1 teaspoon sea salt

1 teaspoon freshly ground black pepper

1 teaspoon onion powder

1 teaspoon paprika

½ teaspoon garlic powder

½ teaspoon cayenne pepper

2 large eggs

2 pounds cod, cut into thick strips

1 lemon, cut into wedges

1. Preheat the oven to 450°F.

2. Line 2 baking sheets with aluminum foil and set aside.

3. In a medium bowl, toss the parsnip fries with avocado oil until well coated. Evenly spread the parsnips onto one of the foil-lined baking sheets.

4. Bake in the oven for 10 to 15 minutes, until golden brown.

5. Meanwhile, in a shallow bowl mix together the coconut flour, almond flour, salt, pepper, onion powder, paprika, garlic powder, and cayenne pepper. In a separate shallow bowl, whisk the eggs until lightly beaten.

6. Dredge one piece of fish at a time in the flour mixture, then into the eggs, and then back into the flour mixture to coat the fish strips.

7. Put the breaded fish onto the foil-lined baking sheet in a single layer and repeat with the remaining fish. Bake for 10 to 12 minutes, flipping half-way through.

8. Divide the fish, fries, and lemon wedges into 2 containers.

STORAGE: Once cooled, store in covered containers in the refrigerator for up to 3 days. To reheat, microwave for 2 to 3 minutes or bake in a 400°F oven for 8 to 10 minutes. Store in freezer-safe containers for up to 1 month. To defrost, refrigerate overnight and follow reheat instructions.

SMART SHOPPING: If fresh cod is not readily available at your local market, opt for frozen fish and thaw before cooking.

Per Serving (1 container): Calories: 921; Fat: 38g; Protein: 112g; Total Carbs: 39g; Fiber: 17g; Sodium: 1904mg; Iron: 4g

Chicken and Veggie Fried Cauliflower Rice

Serves 4 — Prep time: 35 minutes — Cook time: 30 minutes

Fried rice has always been a personal favorite, and this version has all the flavors I love but is packed with veggies. For this recipe I use my go-to Cauliflower Rice (page 95) recipe as the base and then pile on more veggies and lean protein. Despite the sneaky veggies, this dish looks and tastes like the original. And just like the original, you can easily swap out the chicken for pork, beef, or shrimp—or omit the protein altogether for a meatless option.

Cauliflower Rice (page 95)

1 egg

2 tablespoons coconut flour

½ teaspoon sea salt

½ teaspoon freshly ground black pepper

3 tablespoons sesame oil

1 pound boneless chicken breasts, diced

½ onion, minced

2 garlic cloves, minced

½ cup peas

1 carrot, peeled and diced

3 tablespoons coconut aminos

1. Prepare the cauliflower rice and set aside.
2. In a large mixing bowl, stir together the cauliflower rice, egg, coconut flour, salt, and pepper. Set aside.
3. In a large skillet, heat the oil over medium-high heat.
4. Carefully place the chicken in the skillet and cook for 8 minutes, until browned.
5. Once the chicken is cooked through, add the onion and garlic. Cook for about 60 seconds, until fragrant.
6. Add the cauliflower rice mixture, peas, carrot, and coconut aminos to the same skillet, and stir to combine all ingredients. Sauté for 10 minutes.
7. Divide the fried rice evenly between 4 containers.

STORAGE: Once cooled, store in covered containers in the refrigerator for up to 5 days. To reheat, microwave for 2 to 3 minutes.

SMART SHOPPING: Streamline your grocery list and prep by opting for frozen veggies in place of fresh.

Per Serving (1 container): Calories: 378; Fat: 19g; Protein: 32g; Total Carbs: 20g; Fiber: 6g; Sodium: 777mg; Iron: 2g

Thai Basil Beef and Noodles

Serves 4 — Prep time: 15 minutes — Cook time: 20 minutes

This is not your typical weeknight meal unless you are reaching for the takeout menu. While traditional Thai Basil Beef calls for Thai basil, I find that you can still pack in all the flavor with Italian basil, which is more commonly available. By prepping this recipe over the weekend, you can enjoy all of the bold flavors of Thai Basil Beef and Noodles in minutes—less time than it would take to place an order.

2 pounds flank steak, thinly sliced

2 teaspoons arrowroot flour

3 tablespoons extra-virgin olive oil, divided

Sea salt

4 garlic cloves, minced

½ white onion, sliced

2 red bell peppers, sliced

2 Thai chiles, sliced

¼ cup coconut aminos

1 tablespoon fish sauce

1 cup fresh basil leaves

2 zucchinis, spiralized into noodles

1. In a large mixing bowl, combine the steak, arrowroot flour, and 1 tablespoon olive oil. Season with salt and toss until evenly coated.

2. In a large skillet, heat the remaining oil over high heat.

3. Add half of the steak to the skillet and cook for 2 to 3 minutes per side, until well browned. Repeat with the remaining steak.

4. Remove the steak from the skillet and reduce the heat to medium. Add the garlic to the skillet and cook for 30 seconds, until fragrant. Add the onion, red bell peppers, and chiles. Season with salt and cook for 5 to 7 minutes, until onions are tender.

5. Add the steak back into the skillet. Add the coconut aminos and fish sauce. Let simmer for 2 to 3 minutes, until the sauce reduces and thickens.

CONTINUED

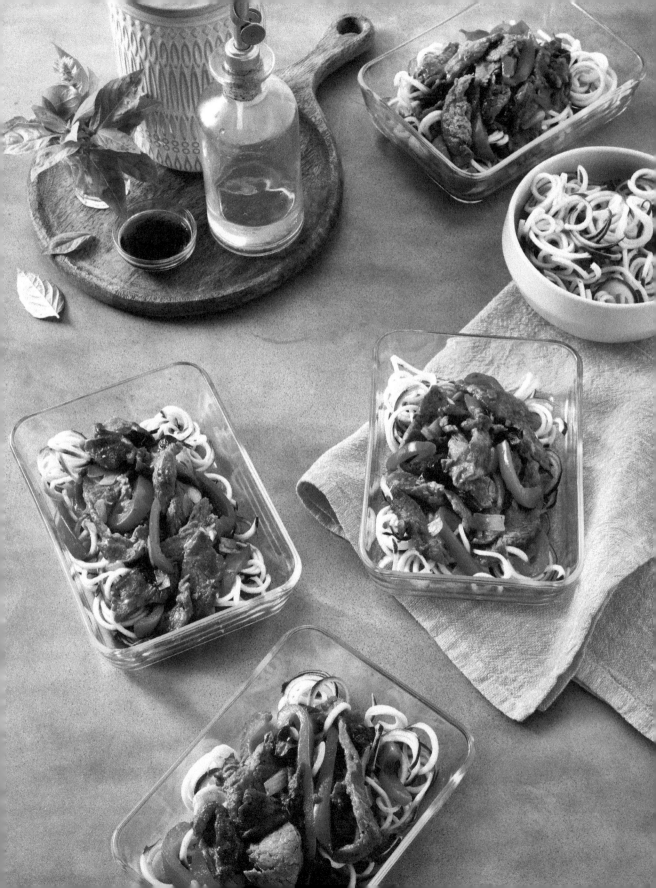

Thai Basil Beef and Noodles

CONTINUED

6. Remove the skillet from the stove and stir in the basil until wilted.

7. Divide the zucchini noodles evenly between 4 containers. Divide the steak and veggies between the 4 containers on top of the noodles.

STORAGE: Once cooled, store in covered containers in the refrigerator for up to 5 days. To reheat, microwave for 2 to 3 minutes.

SIMPLE SWAP: If you cannot find Thai chiles at the local market, simply swap for ¼ teaspoon of red pepper flakes.

Per Serving (1 container): Calories: 572; Fat: 21g; Protein: 71g; Total Carbs: 25g; Fiber: 3g; Sodium: 1398mg; Iron: 8g

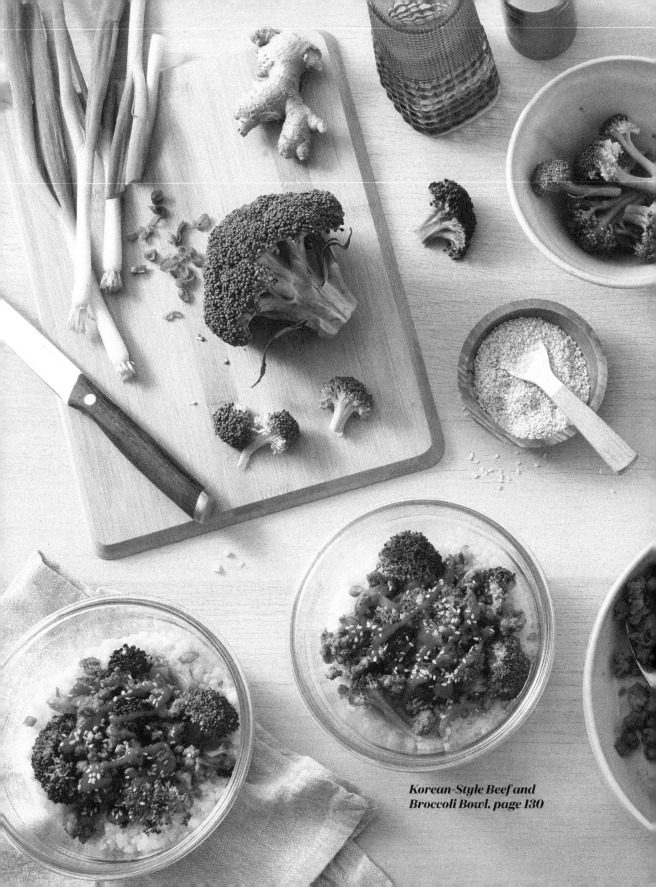

Korean-Style Beef and Broccoli Bowl, page 130

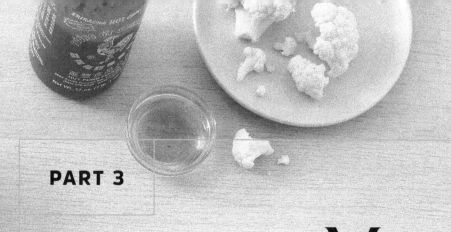

PART 3

More Prep-Friendly Paleo Recipes

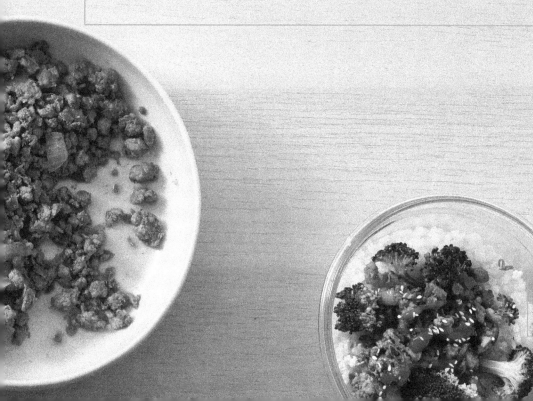

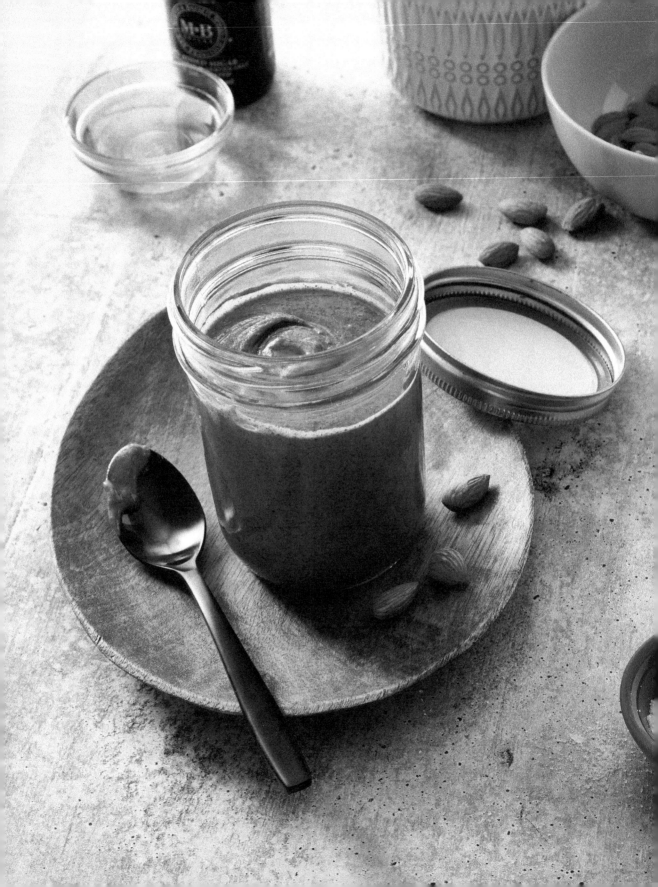

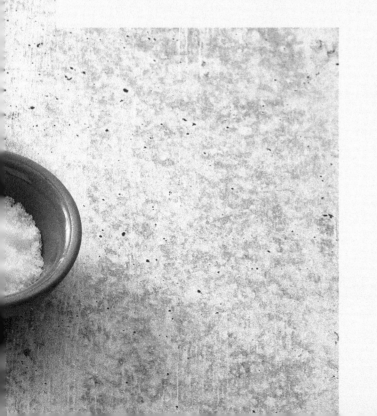

Staples

Tzatziki

Makes 1 cup — Prep time: 15 minutes

Tzatziki is made with just a few simple ingredients, and this version replaces traditional yogurt with coconut milk yogurt. Refreshing cucumber and zingy lemon make it the perfect condiment for just about everything. Spoon it onto an entrée or serve on its own as a tasty dip with fresh veggies. I like to drizzle mine with olive oil and crack a little fresh pepper on top.

1 cup plain, unsweetened coconut milk yogurt

¼ cucumber, grated

2 garlic cloves, minced

2 tablespoons finely chopped fresh dill

1 tablespoon freshly squeezed lemon juice

½ tablespoon extra-virgin olive oil

Sea salt

Freshly ground black pepper

1. In a mixing bowl, combine coconut yogurt, cucumber, garlic, dill, lemon juice, and olive oil. Season with salt and pepper and stir until well combined.

2. Taste and adjust the seasoning as needed.

3. Transfer the tzatziki to a mason jar or other storage container with a lid.

STORAGE: Store in the refrigerator for 5 to 7 days.

SMART SHOPPING: I recommend using an unsweetened Greek-style coconut milk yogurt like CocoYo, or unsweetened Greek-style almond milk yogurt such as Kite Hill.

COOKING HACK: Make sure your grated cucumber is well drained. Place the grated cucumber in the middle of a cheesecloth, tea towel, or fine mesh sieve. Lightly salt the cucumber to pull excess moisture from the fruit, then twist the cloth/towel or push against the sieve to drain the fruit.

Per Serving (¼ cup): Calories: 47; Fat: 4g; Protein: 0g; Total Carbs: 4g; Fiber: 1g; Sodium: 51mg; Iron: 0g

Almond Butter

Makes 2 cups — Prep time: 15 minutes — Cook time: 10 minutes

Homemade almond butter sounds intimidating, but it is relatively easy to whip up and may be even tastier than store bought. Not to mention, it only really takes two simple ingredients. In this recipe I add a little bit of maple syrup for sweetness and vanilla to balance the flavor. You can modify this recipe by swapping the almonds for peanuts, cashews, or pecans, or add spices like cinnamon and nutmeg for extra flavor. I enjoy almond butter with fresh fruit and spread it on top of my Banana Bread (page 100).

3 cups raw almonds

Pinch of sea salt

2 tablespoons maple syrup (optional)

½ teaspoon vanilla extract (optional)

1. Preheat the oven to 350°F and line a baking sheet with parchment paper.

2. Arrange the almonds on the baking sheet in a single layer and cook for 10 minutes, tossing halfway through.

3. Transfer the almonds to a food processor and blend until creamy, stopping to scrape down the sides with a spatula as needed. If the mixture gets hot along the way, stop and let it cool for a few minutes.

4. Once the almond butter is smooth and creamy, add the salt, maple syrup, and vanilla extract (if using) until evenly mixed.

5. Let cool and then transfer the almond butter to a mason jar or other storage container with a lid.

STORAGE: Store in the refrigerator for up to 2 weeks.

COOKING HACK: Cut down on prep by opting for roasted almonds in place of raw and skip the roasting step in this recipe.

Per Serving (2 tablespoons): Calories: 141; Fat: 12g; Protein: 5g; Total Carbs: 5g; Fiber: 3g; Sodium: 10mg; Iron: 1g

Taco Seasoning

Makes ½ cup — Prep time: 5 minutes

Store-bought seasoning can be loaded with additives, and the flavor doesn't hold a candle to this homemade version. All of the spices used in this recipe are everyday pantry items, so you likely have all of the ingredients you need. This versatile mix can be used for more than just ground beef and turkey in tacos and burritos. Try sprinkling it on chicken, fish, and more!

4 tablespoons chili powder

2 tablespoons ground cumin

1 tablespoon paprika

2 teaspoons onion powder

2 teaspoons garlic powder

1 teaspoon dried oregano

½ teaspoon sea salt

½ teaspoon red pepper flakes

1. In a mixing bowl, stir together the chili powder, cumin, paprika, onion powder, garlic powder, oregano, salt, and red pepper flakes until thoroughly combined.
2. Transfer the taco seasoning to an airtight container.

STORAGE: Store in an airtight container for up to 30 days.

COOKING HACK: For best results, use 2 tablespoons of the seasoning mixed with ¼ cup of water per 1 pound of meat.

Per Serving (2 tablespoons): Calories: 49; Fat: 2g; Protein: 2g; Total Carbs: 9g; Fiber: 4g; Sodium: 532mg; Iron: 4g

Marinara Sauce

Makes 3 cups — Prep time: 10 minutes — Cook time: 25 minutes

Store-bought tomato sauce can lack flavor and is often full of sugar. This simple yet classic marinara sauce is our go-to in place of store bought. It's full of flavor and super easy to prepare, with no chopping required. This sauce is perfect on top of zucchini noodles or your favorite gluten-free pasta. It also makes the perfect pizza sauce.

¼ cup extra-virgin olive oil

6 garlic cloves, minced

1 tablespoon tomato paste

1 (28-ounce) can crushed tomatoes

1 cup water

½ teaspoon sea salt

½ teaspoon black pepper

1 teaspoon dried basil

1 teaspoon dried oregano

½ teaspoon onion powder

¼ teaspoon red pepper flakes

1 cup chopped fresh basil

1. In a large pot, heat the oil over medium-high heat.

2. Add the garlic and cook for 1 minute, stirring occasionally.

3. Add the tomato paste to the pot and cook for another minute.

4. Add the crushed tomatoes, water, herbs and spices to the pot, reserving the fresh basil.

5. When the sauce begins to boil, reduce heat to low and let simmer for 15 to 20 minutes until the sauce thickens.

6. Stir in the fresh basil.

7. Let cool and then transfer the sauce to a mason jar or other storage container with a lid.

STORAGE: Store in the refrigerator for up to 5 days. To reheat, microwave for 2 to 3 minutes. Alternately, you can store in the freezer for 1 to 2 months. To reheat, thaw and warm on the stove with a little olive oil.

COOKING HACK: If you are looking to balance the acidity of the tomatoes in the marinara sauce, try adding a pinch of coconut sugar.

Per Serving (½ cup): Calories: 46; Fat: 0g; Protein: 3g; Total Carbs: 10g; Fiber: 3g; Sodium: 443mg; Iron: 2g

Pesto Sauce

Makes 1 cup — Prep time: 5 minutes

While traditional pesto sauce includes parmesan cheese, this version is dairy-free but packed with flavor! With just 6 simple ingredients and 5 minutes, this recipe is quick and easy to whip up. There are so many ways to enjoy this sauce. Try stirring a dollop into a bowl of zoodles, spread it on top of crackers, or use it as a replacement for red sauce in your favorite recipe.

4 cups fresh basil leaves, packed

½ cup pine nuts, lightly toasted

3 garlic cloves, chopped

Sea salt

½ cup extra-virgin olive oil

2 teaspoons freshly squeezed lemon juice

1. In a food processor, combine the basil, pine nuts, and garlic, and season with salt.
2. Turn the processor on and slowly add the olive oil and lemon juice until the ingredients are fully combined.
3. Transfer the pesto to a mason jar or other storage container with a lid.

STORAGE: Store in the refrigerator for up to 5 days.

SIMPLE SWAP: For a twist on this traditional dairy-free pesto recipe, swap the basil for spinach and the pine nuts for shelled walnuts.

Per Serving (2 tablespoons): Calories: 179; Fat: 19g; Protein: 2g; Total Carbs: 3g; Fiber: 1g; Sodium: 27mg; Iron: 1g

Cauliflower Rice

Serves 4 — Prep time: 10 minutes — Cook time: 15 minutes

Cauliflower is the Swiss Army knife of vegetables. It can be transformed into pizza crust, pureed into a starchy mash, covered in buffalo sauce in place of chicken wings, and riced to replace rice and grains in just about any meal. I use cauliflower rice as the base for burrito bowls, tossed with veggies for a fried rice, and in my Paleo tabbouleh. If you are serving cauliflower rice as a side, kick up the flavor by adding ½ teaspoon of onion powder, ⅓ cup of cilantro, and the juice of 1 lime.

1 head cauliflower, trimmed into florets

1 tablespoon extra-virgin olive oil

1 garlic clove

Sea salt

Freshly ground black pepper

1. Pulse the cauliflower florets in a food processor until the cauliflower is a fine, rice-like consistency.

2. In a large skillet over medium heat, heat the olive oil. Add the garlic and cook for 30 seconds, until fragrant.

3. Add the cauliflower and season with salt and pepper. Cook for 10 to 12 minutes, stirring frequently.

4. Divide the cauliflower into 4 containers.

STORAGE: Once cooled, store in covered containers in the refrigerator for up to 5 days. To reheat, microwave for 1 to 2 minutes. Alternately, you can store in the freezer for 1 to 2 months. To reheat, thaw and warm on the stove with a little olive oil.

COOKING HACK: If you don't have a food processor, you can use a box grater to get a similar, fine rice consistency. You can also find pre-riced cauliflower (fresh or frozen) in most grocery stores.

Per Serving (1 container): Calories: 68; Fat: 4g; Protein: 3g; Total Carbs: 8g; Fiber: 3g; Sodium: 83mg; Iron: 1g

Mashed Cauliflower

Serves 4 — Prep time: 10 minutes — Cook time: 10 minutes

In addition to being converted into rice, cauliflower is also the base of this easy recipe. Made with just 4 simple ingredients, this creamy cauliflower puree makes a delicious side dish and is the perfect alternative to mashed potatoes. Not only is this a way to sneak extra veggies into your diet, but it also has a delicious, deep nutty flavor. Spice up this recipe by adding roasted garlic and 1 teaspoon of fresh rosemary or thyme.

1 teaspoon sea salt, plus more for seasoning water

1 large head cauliflower, trimmed into florets

2 tablespoons extra-virgin olive oil

Freshly ground black pepper

1. Bring a large pot of water to a boil over high heat. Add a large pinch of salt.

2. Add the cauliflower to the pot and cook for 10 minutes. The cauliflower will be very tender.

3. Drain the florets, reserving ¼ cup of the water in a small dish.

4. In a food processor, puree the cauliflower, slowly pouring in the olive oil and reserved water until smooth. Scrape down the sides of the food processor with a spatula as needed to incorporate all the cauliflower.

5. Season with salt and pepper.

6. Divide the cauliflower into 4 containers.

STORAGE: Once cooled, store in covered containers in the refrigerator for up to 5 days. To reheat, microwave for 2 to 3 minutes.

COOKING HACK: The key is to salt the water generously to add flavor while cooking. I recommend using about 2 heaping teaspoons of sea salt for each quart of water.

Per Serving (1 container): Calories: 112; Fat: 7g; Protein: 4g; Total Carbs: 11g; Fiber: 4g; Sodium: 653mg; Iron: 1g

Egg Wraps

Makes 5 wraps — Prep time: 10 minutes — Cook time: 10 minutes

When I first gave up gluten and grains, it was difficult to find a substitute for wraps, breads, and bagels so that I could enjoy sandwiches, burritos, and more. Luckily, I was inspired to create an egg-based wrap that I use for everything from Breakfast Tacos (page 79) to burritos and wraps! Keep a handful of these wraps in the refrigerator and use them to prep breakfast and lunch. You can even spread some almond butter and dark chocolate on one of these wraps for a tasty dessert.

1 tablespoon avocado oil

5 eggs

1. In a small skillet, heat the avocado oil over medium heat.
2. In a bowl, crack 1 egg and whisk well.
3. Pour the egg into the pan and tilt the pan to spread the egg into a large circle on the bottom of the pan.
4. Let the egg cook for 30 seconds on one side. Carefully flip the egg with a large spatula and let cook another 30 seconds.
5. Remove the wrap from the pan and repeat steps 2 through 4 with the remaining eggs.
6. Divide the egg wraps into 5 containers or plastic bags, or store in one container, separating each wrap with parchment paper.

STORAGE: Once cooled, store in covered containers in the refrigerator for up to 5 days. To reheat, microwave for 30 to 60 seconds.

COOKING HACK: To amp up the flavor of the egg wraps, season with sea salt, freshly ground black pepper, paprika, basil, or any mixture of your favorite spices or herbs.

Per Serving (1 egg wrap): Calories: 92; Fat: 7g; Protein: 6g; Total Carbs: 1g; Fiber: 0g; Sodium: 55mg; Iron: 1g

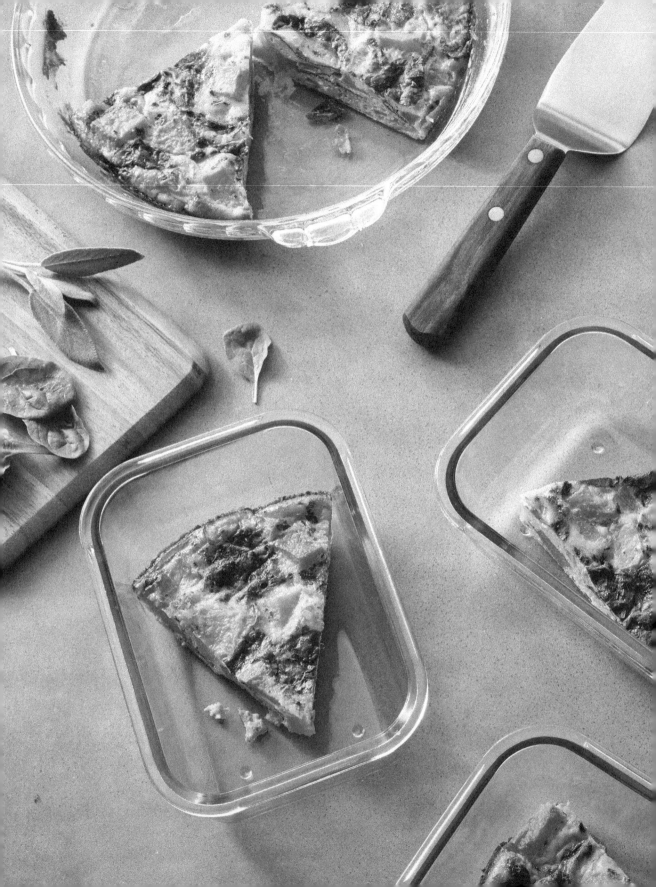

Breakfasts

Banana Bread

Serves 5 — Prep time: 10 minutes — Cook time: 40 minutes

This is a gluten- and dairy-free version of classic banana bread, sweetened with unrefined sugar and perfectly moist. The warm cinnamon and nutmeg not only lend to the flavor, but also fill the house with a delicious smell. You can enjoy this bread plain, or even add chopped walnuts or chocolate chips!

¼ cup coconut oil, plus more for greasing

3 eggs

2 tablespoons maple syrup

1 teaspoon vanilla extract

1½ cups almond flour

½ teaspoon cinnamon

½ teaspoon nutmeg

1 teaspoon baking powder

1 teaspoon baking soda

½ teaspoon sea salt

3 ripe bananas, mashed

1. Preheat the oven to 375°F and grease a loaf pan with coconut oil.
2. In a medium mixing bowl, whisk together the eggs, coconut oil, maple syrup, and vanilla extract.
3. In a separate mixing bowl, combine the almond flour, cinnamon, nutmeg, baking powder, baking soda, and salt.
4. Add the dry ingredients to the wet, and mix well. Add the mashed banana and mix until just combined.
5. Pour the batter into the prepared loaf pan and bake for about 40 minutes, until golden brown.
6. Let cool and then slice it into 5 large slices or 10 small slices.
7. Divide the slices between 5 containers.

STORAGE: Once cooled, store in covered containers in the refrigerator for up to 5 days.

COOKING HACK: Transform this delicious banana bread into indulgent French Toast! Simply whisk together eggs, coconut milk, vanilla extract, and cinnamon in a shallow bowl. Dip a slice of the banana bread into the egg mixture and then cook on an oiled skillet for 2 to 3 minutes per side.

Per Serving (1 container): Calories: 443; Fat: 34g; Protein: 11g; Total Carbs: 29g; Fiber: 6g; Sodium: 623mg; Iron: 2g

Bacon-Wrapped Egg Cups

Serves 5 — Prep time: 10 minutes — Cook time: 25 minutes

Egg cups make for a delicious start to the day or an equally tasty snack! Whip up a batch or double and store half in the freezer so you have them on hand. You can also switch things up by adding diced jalapeño, or swapping the bell pepper for another veggie. Diced sweet potato and broccoli both work well.

Coconut oil, for greasing

10 strips bacon

1 small red bell pepper, finely chopped

10 large eggs

Sea salt

Freshly ground black pepper

1. Preheat the oven to 400°F. Meanwhile, grease 10 cups of a muffin tin with coconut oil.

2. Wrap 1 piece of bacon around the inside of each cup. Divide the bell pepper evenly between the cups.

3. Bake for 10 to 12 minutes, until the bacon fat starts to render and the bacon begins to turn light brown on the top edges.

4. Remove the muffin tin from the oven and crack an egg into each cup.

5. Continue baking for about 10 minutes, until the bacon is crisp, the egg whites are cooked through, and the yolks are still runny. Season with salt and pepper.

6. Let the egg cups cool for a few minutes, then run a butter knife around the edges of each cup and remove.

7. Divide the egg cups between 5 containers.

STORAGE: Once cooled, store in covered containers in the refrigerator for up to 5 days. To reheat egg cups, microwave for 25 to 30 seconds, or in increments of 15 seconds to avoid rubbery eggs.

COOKING HACK: For extra creamy eggs, whisk the eggs with a tablespoon of almond milk.

Per Serving (2 egg cups): Calories: 242; Fat: 17g; Protein: 18g; Total Carbs: 2g; Fiber: 0g; Sodium: 425mg; Iron: 1g

Butternut Squash and Apple Hash with Eggs

Serves 5 — Prep time: 15 minutes — Cook time: 35 minutes

This hearty hash is a delicious and satisfying way to start the day. In this recipe the tender root veggies, crisp apple, and smoky bacon play together for the perfect combination in every bite. You can also stir in spinach or kale for an extra serving of greens. I like to top the hash with a fried egg, but you can make it your own with poached or scrambled eggs, if you prefer.

6 slices bacon, chopped

1 yellow onion, diced

1 small butternut squash, peeled and chopped

1 apple, diced

1 tablespoon extra-virgin olive oil

5 eggs

Sea salt

Freshly ground black pepper

1. Heat a large skillet over medium heat. Add the bacon and cook, stirring occasionally, until crisp, about 5 minutes. Remove with a slotted spoon and set aside.

2. Add the onion to the skillet and cook until translucent, about 3 to 5 minutes. Add the butternut squash to the skillet and spread it out evenly until it starts to brown, about 10 minutes, stirring occasionally.

3. When the butternut squash is golden brown, add the apple, and cook until it begins to soften, about 5 to 8 minutes.

4. Meanwhile, in a small nonstick skillet, heat the olive oil over medium heat. Crack one egg into the pan and cook for 3 minutes, or until the egg white is set. Flip the egg and cook 1 minute more. Remove from pan, season with salt and pepper, and set aside. Repeat with the remaining eggs.

5. Divide the butternut squash hash across 5 containers, and add 1 egg on top of each hash.

STORAGE: Once cooled, store in covered containers in the refrigerator for up to 5 days. To reheat, remove the egg and microwave for 2 to 3 minutes. Add the egg and reheat for an additional 15 to 30 seconds.

SIMPLE SWAP: A lot of Paleo breakfast recipes rely on eggs as a source of protein, but you can skip the eggs altogether. Another great option is pairing this hash with ground turkey or beef, or my Spicy Sausage Patties (page 58).

SMART SHOPPING: Butternut squash is available year-round, but is best fall through winter. When choosing a squash, look for one that feels heavy for its size with a fat neck and small bulb, as it will yield the most meat.

Per Serving (1 container): Calories: 201; Fat: 11g; Protein: 10g; Total Carbs: 17g; Fiber: 4g; Sodium: 252mg; Iron: 1g

Brussels Sprouts and Bacon Egg Bake

Serves 5 — Prep time: 15 minutes — Cook time: 1 hour 10 minutes

This hearty egg bake is loaded with tender sweet potatoes and Brussels sprouts, but you can easily swap out them out with your favorite vegetables to switch things up. Roasting root veggies in advance ensures that they will be tender in the casserole, but if you are working with softer veggies, you don't need to roast them first.

Coconut oil, for greasing

1 sweet potato, peeled and diced

1 cup Brussels sprouts, trimmed and halved

2 tablespoons extra-virgin olive oil

Sea salt

6 slices bacon, chopped

½ onion, diced

6 eggs

2½ tablespoons full-fat coconut milk

¼ teaspoon garlic powder

Freshly ground black pepper

1. Preheat the oven to 400°F. Meanwhile, grease a 9-by-9-inch casserole dish with coconut oil, and line a baking sheet with parchment paper.

2. Arrange the sweet potato and Brussels sprouts on the baking sheet and drizzle with the olive oil. Toss to coat well and season with salt. Arrange the vegetables in a single layer on the baking sheet and bake for 20 minutes, or until they are golden brown and crisp.

3. While the vegetables roast, heat a large skillet over medium-high heat. Cook the bacon, stirring occasionally, until crisp, about 5 minutes. Remove with a slotted spoon and set aside.

4. Lower the heat to medium-low and add the onion to the skillet. Cook, stirring occasionally, for about 20 minutes, until the onion is caramelized.

5. Meanwhile, in a medium mixing bowl combine the eggs, milk, and garlic powder. Season with salt and pepper and whisk well.

6. Lower the oven temperature to 375°F. Add the sweet potatoes, Brussels sprouts, caramelized onions, and bacon to your casserole dish. Pour the egg mixture over the vegetables.

7. Bake for 25 minutes, until the center is set and the edges are light brown. Remove and let cool.

8. Divide the casserole between 5 containers.

STORAGE: Once cooled, store in covered containers in the refrigerator for up to 5 days. To reheat, microwave for 1 to 2 minutes.

COOKING HACK: When roasting vegetables, you need to evenly coat them in oil so they cook and crisp evenly. This can be done in a mixing bowl; however, I like not having to wash another a dish and instead toss the vegetables directly on the pan with tongs.

Per Serving (1 container): Calories: 235; Fat: 17g; Protein: 11g; Total Carbs: 9g; Fiber: 2g; Sodium: 278mg; Iron: 1g

Caramelized Onion and Spinach Frittata

Serves 5 — Prep time: 15 minutes — Cook time: 1 hour

The only thing better than a savory breakfast is a savory breakfast that is already made and requires no effort during the week. I love that this frittata feels like a treat but requires very little prep in order to enjoy it any (or every) day of the week. In fact, this dish would also be delicious for lunch or dinner.

1 tablespoon extra-virgin olive oil

½ yellow onion, diced

½ small butternut squash, cubed

6 eggs

½ teaspoon sea salt, plus more for seasoning

⅓ cup unsweetened almond milk

1 teaspoon dried sage

¼ teaspoon dried thyme

½ teaspoon dried parsley

1 cup packed spinach

1. Preheat the oven to 400°F and line a baking sheet with parchment paper.

2. In a large skillet, heat the olive oil over medium heat. Add the onion to the skillet. Cook, stirring occasionally, for about 20 minutes, until it is caramelized.

3. Meanwhile, arrange the butternut squash on the baking sheet and drizzle with the remaining oil. Toss to coat well and season with salt. Bake for 15 minutes.

4. Meanwhile in a large mixing bowl, combine eggs, almond milk, sage, thyme, parsley, and salt. Add the spinach, caramelized onions, and cooked butternut squash and stir to combine.

5. Lower the oven temperature to 375°F. Pour the mixture into a 9-inch glass pie dish.

6. Bake for 30 minutes, until the center is set.

7. Divide the frittata between 5 containers.

STORAGE: Once cooled, store in covered containers in the refrigerator for up to 5 days. To reheat, microwave for 2 to 3 minutes.

SIMPLE SWAP: While I love using fresh vegetables and greens in my recipes, sometimes the market is out of what you are looking for and the options don't look great. That is why I always keep frozen veggies and greens in my freezer. In this recipe you can swap 1 cup of packed fresh spinach for ½ cup of well-drained frozen spinach. You can also swap spinach for kale or another green of your choice.

Per Serving (1 container): Calories: 133; Fat: 9g; Protein: 8g; Total Carbs: 7g; Fiber: 2g; Sodium: 320mg; Iron: 1g

Spinach and Artichoke Egg Bake

Serves 5 — Prep time: 15 minutes — Cook time: 30 minutes

This breakfast casserole was inspired by one of my all-time favorite appetizers. Here I have transformed classic spinach and artichoke dip into an easy-to-prep breakfast dish that is sure to make it into your weekly meal prep rotation. This casserole can also be made for a crowd. Either way I prefer to prep it in advance because it allows the flavors to marinate together.

Coconut oil, for greasing

6 large eggs

2 large egg whites

¼ cup unsweetened almond milk

1 teaspoon dried tarragon

Sea salt

Freshly ground black pepper

1 cup packed spinach

¼ cup scallions, finely chopped

½ cup chopped canned artichoke hearts, drained and patted dry

¼ cup red bell pepper, diced

1 clove garlic, minced

1. Preheat the oven to 375°F, and grease a 9-by-9-inch casserole dish with coconut oil.

2. In a large mixing bowl, whisk together the eggs, egg whites, almond milk, and tarragon. Season with salt and pepper. Fold in the spinach, scallions, artichokes, red bell pepper, and garlic.

3. Pour the mixture into the casserole dish.

4. Bake for 25 to 30 minutes, until the center is set.

5. Divide the quiche between 5 containers.

STORAGE: Once cooled, store in covered containers in the refrigerator for up to 5 days. To reheat, microwave for 2 to 3 minutes.

SIMPLE SWAP: In this recipe, along with many others throughout the book, you can swap the almond milk for coconut milk.

Per Serving (1 container): Calories: 142; Fat: 9g; Protein: 10g; Total Carbs: 4g; Fiber: 1g; Sodium: 190mg; Iron: 1g

Southwest Breakfast Casserole

Serves 5 — Prep time: 15 minutes — Cook time: 50 minutes

Breakfast casseroles are a great meal prep option because they are easy to make and hold up well throughout the week. A breakfast casserole is also an excellent opportunity to use up any leftover vegetables. The key to the perfect egg casserole is to have a variety of textures. The crispy bacon, diced peppers, and shredded sweet potatoes all offer something a little different in this dish.

Coconut oil, for greasing

6 slices bacon

8 eggs

½ cup unsweetened almond milk

½ teaspoon chili powder

½ teaspoon ground cumin

¼ teaspoon sea salt

1 sweet potato, peeled and shredded

1 red bell pepper, diced

1 jalapeño pepper, finely diced

1. Preheat the oven to 375°F. Line a baking sheet with parchment paper and grease a 9-by-9-inch casserole dish with coconut oil.

2. Arrange the bacon on the baking sheet and cook for 15 minutes, or until crisp.

3. Meanwhile in a large mixing bowl, whisk together the eggs, almond milk, chili powder, cumin, and salt. Fold in the sweet potatoes, bell pepper, and jalapeño.

4. Roughly chop the bacon and add it to the mixture.

5. Pour the mixture into the casserole dish. Bake for 30 to 35 minutes, until the center is set.

6. Divide the casserole between 5 containers.

STORAGE: Once cooled, store in covered containers in the refrigerator for up to 5 days. To reheat, microwave for 2 to 3 minutes.

COOKING HACK: The seeds and inner membranes of a jalapeño often hold the most heat. To adjust the heat level of this recipe, remove the seeds and membrane before dicing the jalapeño.

Per Serving (1 container): Calories: 213; Fat: 14g; Protein: 13g; Total Carbs: 8g; Fiber: 2g; Sodium: 407mg; Iron: 1g

Sausage-Stuffed Breakfast Sweet Potatoes

Serves 4 — Prep time: 20 minutes — Cook time: 1 hour

Stuffed vegetables have been a trend for quite a while, from peppers and avocados to mushrooms and zucchini boats. This recipe is a twist on a twice-baked potato for breakfast. Once you master this version, you can put your own twist on this tasty dish. Try adding a green, like kale or spinach. Top with diced avocado. Or go for a completely different flavor profile by omitting the eggs and sausage in place of fresh fruit and nut butter.

2 sweet potatoes

1 tablespoon extra-virgin olive oil

1 pound ground turkey

½ teaspoon sea salt

¼ teaspoon freshly ground black pepper

¾ teaspoon ground sage

¾ teaspoon thyme

¼ teaspoon marjoram

¼ teaspoon red pepper flakes

6 eggs

¼ cup full-fat coconut milk

1. Preheat the oven to 400°F and line a baking sheet with parchment paper.

2. Poke 4 holes in both sweet potatoes with a knife and place the sweet potatoes on the baking sheet. Cook for 1 hour, until soft.

3. Meanwhile, heat the oil in a large skillet over medium-high heat. Add the ground turkey and cook for 5 to 8 minutes, until brown. Add the salt, pepper, sage, thyme, marjoram, and red pepper flakes and stir until well combined. Remove the turkey from the skillet with a slotted spoon.

4. In a large mixing bowl, whisk together the eggs and coconut milk. Pour the egg mixture in the skillet and cook for 2 to 3 minutes, stirring consistently for fluffy eggs.

5. When the sweet potatoes are cooked, let them cool. Halve the sweet potato and remove the flesh from the middle of each half, creating a well.

6. In a large mixing bowl, mash the sweet potato flesh. Then fold in the scrambled eggs and turkey.

7. Evenly divide the egg mixture between each of the sweet potato halves.

8. Into 4 containers, place one sweet potato half each.

STORAGE: Once cooled, store in covered containers in the refrigerator for up to 5 days. To reheat, microwave for 2 to 3 minutes.

COOKING HACK: Roasting the sweet potatoes in the oven allows them to develop a rich, sweet flavor. If you are in a pinch and want to speed up prep, simply opt for the microwave instead of the oven. Wash your potato and poke a few holes like the recipe calls for, then cook the potato in the microwave for 5 to 6 minutes, until tender. Be sure to remove with an oven mitt as the potato will be hot!

Per Serving (1 container): Calories: 433; Fat: 24g; Protein: 40g; Total Carbs: 14g; Fiber: 2g; Sodium: 515mg; Iron: 3g

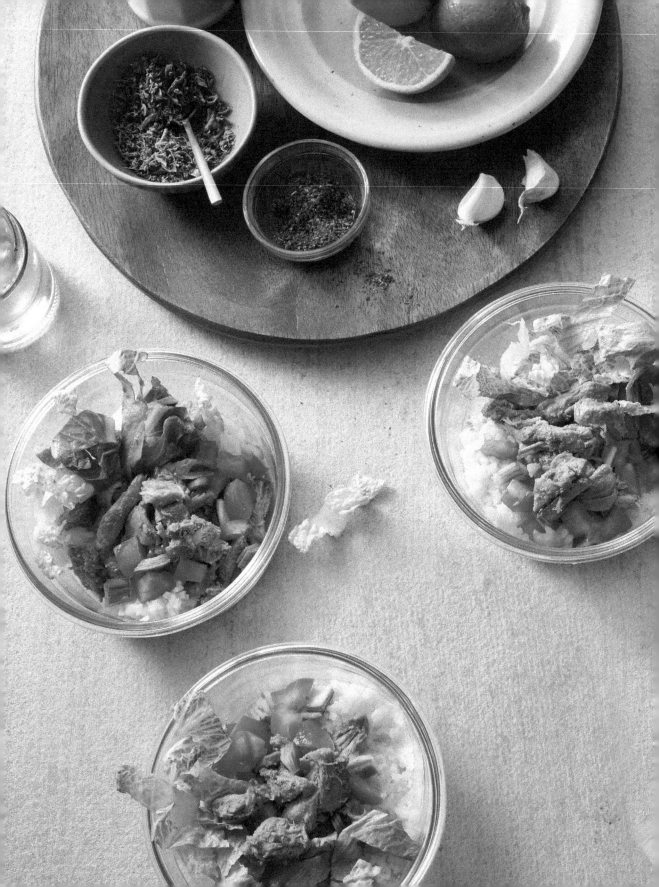

Lunches and Dinners

Buffalo Chicken Salad

Serves 4 — Prep time: 20 minutes — Cook time: 8 minutes

When packing salads in a mason jar, start with the dressing or sauce on the bottom, then move from the heaviest and most nonabsorbent ingredients up through the lighter ingredients until you end up with the salad greens on top. While this salad does not have a dressing, the buffalo sauce is tossed with the chicken before assembling the mason jar. If you opt to serve with a Paleo, dairy-free ranch dressing I recommend keeping it separate in a small cup until you are ready to serve the salad.

2 pounds boneless, skinless chicken breasts

1 cup chicken stock

Sea salt

Freshly ground black pepper

½ cup hot sauce

1 tablespoon grass-fed butter, melted

1 teaspoon apple cider vinegar

Pinch cayenne pepper

1 pint cherry tomatoes, halved

4 celery stalks, chopped

8 bacon slices, cooked and chopped

1 head iceberg lettuce, chopped

1. Put the chicken and chicken stock in a pressure cooker. Season with salt and pepper. Cover the pressure cooker and cook on high pressure for 8 minutes. Once cooking is complete, let pressure release naturally.

2. Carefully remove the pressure lid and shred the chicken with 2 forks.

3. Meanwhile, in a mixing bowl whisk together the hot sauce, butter, apple cider vinegar, and cayenne pepper.

4. Toss the shredded chicken in the buffalo sauce and set aside.

5. Divide the chicken and buffalo sauce between 4 mason jars, then add the tomatoes, celery, bacon, and lettuce.

STORAGE: Once cooled, store covered in the refrigerator for up to 5 days.

SIMPLE SWAP: Swap out the veggies in this salad for your favorites; diced cucumber, onion, and avocado work great. I also love adding shredded cabbage and carrots.

SMART SHOPPING: Hot sauce is made from a base of chile peppers, with salt and vinegar. Look for a version with no added sugar, high-fructose corn syrup, or other unapproved ingredients. Siete Foods and Tessemae's make great Paleo-approved options.

COOKING HACK: If you do not have a pressure cooker, you can make this recipe in a slow cooker. Cook on high for 3 to 4 hours, or low for 6 to 8 hours.

Per Serving (1 container): Calories: 456; Fat: 16g; Protein: 61g; Total Carbs: 15g; Fiber: 5g; Sodium: 1676mg; Iron: 2g

Chicken Cobb Salad

Serves 4 — Prep time: 20 minutes — Cook time: 15 minutes

Colorful rows of vegetables are the mark of a perfectly curated Cobb salad, and this version is arranged artfully in a mason jar to keep your salad from getting soggy. Dressing goes on the bottom, and veggies and other salad goodies get piled on. This order means everything stays separate and dressing-free until you toss the salad together in a bowl to enjoy.

¾ cup extra-virgin olive oil, divided

1 pound boneless, skinless chicken breasts

Sea salt

Freshly ground black pepper

2 tablespoons freshly squeezed lemon juice

2 tablespoons white wine vinegar

1 tablespoon Dijon mustard

4 eggs, hard-boiled and sliced

8 bacon slices, cooked and chopped

1 cucumber, diced

1 cup cherry tomatoes, chopped

1 head romaine lettuce, chopped

1. In a large skillet, heat 1 tablespoon of the olive oil over medium heat.

2. Pat the chicken dry with a paper towel, drizzle with 1 tablespoon of the oil, and season with salt and pepper.

3. Place the chicken in the hot skillet. Cook for 5 to 7 minutes, without moving the chicken, until browned. Flip the chicken and cook for an additional 7 minutes, or until the internal temperature reaches 165°F.

4. Meanwhile, in a mixing bowl combine the lemon juice, vinegar, and Dijon mustard. Slowly whisk in the remaining oil until well combined. Season with salt and pepper.

5. When the chicken is cooked, let it cool and then slice.

6. Divide the lemon vinaigrette between 4 mason jars, and then add the chicken, eggs, bacon, cucumber, tomatoes, and lettuce.

STORAGE: Once cooled, store covered in the refrigerator for up to 5 days.

SIMPLE SWAP: Switch things up by swapping the chicken for salmon, or omit the chicken and bacon altogether for a meatless meal.

Per Serving (1 container): Calories: 723; Fat: 55g; Protein: 49g; Total Carbs: 10g; Fiber: 5g; Sodium: 528mg; Iron: 3g

Chicken Tikka Masala

Serves 4 — Prep time: 40 minutes — Cook time: 2 hours 15 minutes

My husband loves the bold flavors and strong spices that color Indian food, so it came as a no-brainer to recreate his favorite dish, Chicken Tikka Masala, with Paleo-friendly ingredients. I like to prep this recipe before I go on a work trip so that he has something delicious waiting at home that is easy to reheat and enjoy.

Cauliflower Rice (page 95)

2 tablespoons coconut oil

1½ pounds boneless skinless chicken breast, cubed

Sea salt

Freshly ground black pepper

1 yellow onion, diced

4 garlic cloves, minced

1 tablespoon freshly grated ginger or ¼ teaspoon ground ginger

1 (14-ounce) can full-fat coconut milk

2 (14-ounce) cans diced tomatoes

1 tablespoon garam masala

½ teaspoon red pepper flakes

2 tablespoons cilantro, chopped

1. Prepare the cauliflower rice and set aside.

2. In a large skillet, heat the oil over medium heat. Season the chicken with salt and pepper.

3. Add the chicken and cook for about 5 minutes, searing it on all sides. Remove the chicken and set aside.

4. Add the onion, garlic, and ginger to the skillet and sauté for 2 to 3 minutes, until the onion begins to become translucent.

5. Add the coconut milk, tomatoes, garam masala, and red pepper flakes to the skillet. Stir to combine.

6. Add the chicken back to the skillet. Cook for about 5 minutes, until the sauce begins to bubble. Reduce heat to low and let simmer loosely covered for 2 hours, stirring occasionally.

7. Divide the cauliflower rice, chicken, and sauce evenly between 4 containers. Garnish with cilantro.

STORAGE: Once cooled, store in covered containers in the refrigerator for up to 5 days. To reheat, microwave for 2 to 3 minutes.

SIMPLE SWAP: I like using coconut or avocado oil in this recipe, but you can deepen the flavor by replacing the oil with grass-fed butter or ghee.

Per Serving (1 container): Calories: 344; Fat: 16g; Protein: 31g; Total Carbs: 21g; Fiber: 5g; Sodium: 200mg; Iron: 2g

Cashew Chicken and Peppers

Serves 4 — Prep time: 15 minutes — Cook time: 15 minutes

This twist on classic cashew chicken stir-fry features tender chicken, crunchy cashews, and crisp vegetables in a rich sauce. Typically, this type of dish is packed full of ingredients that are off-limits with the Paleo diet; however, with a few simple swaps, I was able to recreate bold flavors in this takeout fake-out. Serve with Cauliflower Rice (page 95) or romaine lettuce and enjoy as lettuce cups.

2 tablespoons extra-virgin olive oil

2 red bell peppers, chopped

2 pounds boneless skinless chicken thighs, chopped

2 tablespoons arrowroot powder

½ teaspoon sea salt

⅓ cup coconut aminos

¼ cup coconut vinegar or apple cider vinegar

2 tablespoons tomato paste

3 tablespoons raw honey

3 garlic cloves, minced

1 tablespoon freshly grated ginger

¼ teaspoon red pepper flakes

1 cup raw cashews

1. In a large skillet, heat the oil over medium heat. Add the bell peppers and sauté for 2 to 3 minutes, until softened.

2. Meanwhile in a mixing bowl, combine the chicken and arrowroot powder. Season with the salt and toss until well coated.

3. Remove the bell peppers from the skillet and set aside. Add the chicken to the skillet and cook for 5 to 8 minutes, stirring frequently.

4. Meanwhile, in a mixing bowl, whisk together the coconut aminos, vinegar, tomato paste, honey, garlic, ginger, and red pepper flakes.

5. Add the sauce to the skillet with the chicken and stir. Add the peppers and cashews to the skillet and continue to stir occasionally. Once the sauce starts to simmer, lower the heat to medium-low, and simmer for 3 to 5 minutes until the sauce thickens.

6. Divide the cashew chicken between 4 containers.

STORAGE: Once cooled, store in covered containers in the refrigerator for up to 5 days. To reheat, microwave for 2 to 3 minutes.

COOKING HACK: Elevate this takeout classic by adding broccoli florets and sliced mushrooms along with the bell pepper.

SIMPLE SWAP: You can swap out 1 tablespoon of freshly grated ginger for ¼ teaspoon of ground ginger. If you can't find coconut vinegar at your grocery store, apple cider vinegar will work as well.

Per Serving (1 container): Calories: 656; Fat: 35g; Protein: 44g; Total Carbs: 45g; Fiber: 3g; Sodium: 1472mg; Iron: 5g

Sweet Potato Chicken Nuggets and Parsnip Fries

Serves 4 — Prep time: 20 minutes — Cook time: 50 minutes

If you are looking to sneak some extra vegetables into your diet, these baked Paleo chicken nuggets are a great option. Easy to prep in advance, they are the perfect make-ahead option for adults and children alike. Here the nuggets are paired with parsnip fries, but roasted broccoli would also work well. Just be sure to serve with a tasty dipping sauce. Double the batch of nuggets and toss half in the freezer for later!

2 large parsnips, peeled and cut into thick fries

4 tablespoons avocado oil, divided

1 pound ground chicken

2 sweet potatoes

2 tablespoons coconut flour

2 scallions, chopped

1 tablespoon garlic powder

1 tablespoon onion powder

1 teaspoon paprika

1 teaspoon sea salt

½ teaspoon black pepper

1. Preheat the oven to 450°F. Line 2 baking sheets with foil and set aside.

2. In a large mixing bowl, toss the parsnips with 2 tablespoons of the avocado oil until well coated. Evenly spread the parsnips onto the foil-lined baking sheets.

3. Bake the parsnips in the oven for 15 to 20 minutes, until golden brown, flipping halfway through.

4. Meanwhile, pulse the sweet potatoes in a food processor until the sweet potato has a fine, rice-like consistency.

5. In a mixing bowl, combine the chicken, sweet potatoes, coconut flour, scallions, garlic powder, onion powder, paprika, sea salt, and black pepper, and mix well. Roll the mixture into 20 nuggets.

6. Remove the parsnip fries from the oven and lightly coat the baking sheets with the remaining oil. Arrange the nuggets on the baking sheets in a single layer.

7. Bake the nuggets in the oven for 25 to 30 minutes, until cooked through, flipping halfway through. Chicken should be 165°F and golden brown.

8. Divide the chicken nuggets and parsnip fries evenly between 4 containers.

STORAGE: Once cooled, store in covered containers in the refrigerator for up to 5 days. To reheat, microwave for 2 to 3 minutes or bake in a 400°F oven for 8 to 10 minutes. Store in freezer-safe containers for up to 1 month. To defrost, refrigerate overnight and follow reheat instructions.

COOKING HACK: If you don't have a food processor, you can use a box grater to get a similar fine-rice consistency. Be sure to watch your fingers while using the grater.

Per Serving (1 container): Calories: 430; Fat: 24g; Protein: 23g; Total Carbs: 33g; Fiber: 8g; Sodium: 713mg; Iron: 2g

Chicken, Spinach, and Tomatoes in Cream Sauce

Serves 4 — Prep time: 10 minutes — Cook time: 25 minutes

This simple one-skillet dish is easy and delicious comfort food at its finest. It makes meal prep and cleanup a breeze! Usually a cream sauce is far from Paleo, but this version is made with rich, full-fat coconut cream. Cooking the sauce in the same pan as the chicken keeps the chicken moist and the sauce flavorful.

4 tablespoons grass-fed butter, divided

4 boneless, skinless chicken breasts

Sea salt

Freshly ground black pepper

1 onion, minced

6 garlic cloves, minced

2 teaspoons oregano

1 jar sun-dried tomatoes, drained and chopped

1 cup chicken broth

1 cup coconut cream

2 cups spinach

1. In a large skillet, heat 2 tablespoons of the butter over medium heat.

2. Pat the chicken dry with a paper towel and season with salt and pepper.

3. Place the chicken in the hot skillet. Cook for 5 to 7 minutes, without moving the chicken, until browned. Flip the chicken and cook for an additional 7 minutes, or until the internal temperature reaches 165°F. Set the chicken aside.

4. Add the remaining butter to the pan to melt. Add the onion, garlic, oregano, and sun-dried tomatoes and sauté for 2 minutes.

5. Add the chicken broth and coconut cream to the skillet and whisk until smooth. Season with salt and pepper.

6. Add the spinach to the pan and cook for 2 to 3 minutes, until wilted, stirring occasionally.

7. Roughly chop the chicken and then add it back to the pan and cook for an additional 3 to 4 minutes.

8. Divide the chicken and sauce evenly between 4 containers.

STORAGE: Once cooled, store in covered containers in the refrigerator for up to 5 days. To reheat, microwave for 2 to 3 minutes.

SIMPLE SWAP: This dish is rich enough to stand on its own, but if you are looking to add in even more veggies, add mushrooms or serve over Mashed Cauliflower (page 96).

Per Serving (1 container): Calories: 783; Fat: 48g; Protein: 69g; Total Carbs: 22g; Fiber: 6g; Sodium: 415mg; Iron: 5g

Skillet Chicken with Tomatoes and Shallots

Serves 4 — Prep time: 15 minutes — Cook time: 1 hour 20 minutes

The title of this recipe does little to describe its bold and delicious flavors, built layer by layer. In one skillet, simple ingredients are cooked one after the other to create a flavorful, succulent chicken dish. Don't be intimidated by the long cook time for this recipe. It is a one-pan meal that is fairly hands-off. Enjoy on its own or serve over Cauliflower Rice (page 95), Mashed Cauliflower (page 96), or roasted vegetables.

8 chicken thighs, bone-in and skin-on

2 tablespoons arrowroot flour

1 tablespoon sea salt

1 tablespoon freshly ground black pepper

2 tablespoons grass-fed butter

10 whole shallots, peeled

2 cups white wine

2 tablespoons Dijon mustard

¼ teaspoon dried tarragon

2 cups cherry tomatoes, quartered

1. Use paper towels to fully dry the chicken thighs and put them on a plate. Sprinkle the flour, salt, and pepper over both sides.

2. In a large, heavy-bottomed skillet, melt the butter over medium-high heat. Once the butter is foamy, add the chicken, 4 thighs at a time, until the skin becomes crispy and brown, about 6 minutes on each side. Remove the chicken thighs and repeat with the remaining pieces, removing all from the pan once browned.

3. Add the shallots to the pan and sauté for 10 minutes, stirring regularly, or until they are soft.

4. Carefully add the wine to deglaze the pan, stirring with a large spoon. Add the mustard and tarragon and stir to combine.

5. Add the chicken thighs back into the pan and cover, cooking over low heat for 30 minutes.

6. After 30 minutes, remove the lid and continue cooking while the sauce thickens, for another 15 to 20 minutes.

7. Add the cherry tomatoes and stir to combine.

8. Divide the chicken, tomatoes, shallots, and sauce evenly between 4 containers.

STORAGE: Once cooled, store in covered containers in the refrigerator for up to 5 days. To reheat, microwave for 3 to 4 minutes.

SMART SHOPPING: Simplify your prep time for this recipe by looking for whole shallots sold already peeled at your local grocery store or market.

Per Serving (1 container): Calories: 1406; Fat: 52g; Protein: 41g; Total Carbs: 33g; Fiber: 4g; Sodium: 3027mg; Iron: 5g

Carnitas Burrito Bowls

Serves 4 — Prep time: 35 minutes — Cook time: 25 minutes

This deconstructed burrito bowl was the first dish I officially meal prepped in advance. In fact, it has been a staple dish in our house since I went Paleo many moons ago. Carnitas is Mexican pulled pork that is succulent and tender thanks to the pressure cooker. Piled on top of cauliflower rice and topped with all of my favorite burrito fillings, this dish is sure to become a regular in your rotation as well.

Cauliflower Rice (page 95)

1 tablespoon extra-virgin olive oil

1 teaspoon chili powder

½ teaspoon dried oregano

½ teaspoon ground cumin

½ teaspoon sea salt

1 pound boneless pork shoulder, chopped into 2-inch pieces

2 medium garlic cloves, minced

2 tomatoes, chopped, divided

½ cup chicken stock

Juice from 1 orange

Juice from 1 lime

½ red onion, diced

1 head romaine lettuce, shredded

1. Prepare the cauliflower rice and set aside.

2. Set the sauté setting on a pressure cooker to high. Put the oil into the cooking pot and allow it to heat up.

3. In a mixing bowl, combine chili powder, dried oregano, ground cumin, and salt. Rub the spice mixture on the pork.

4. Add the seasoned pork shoulder to the cooking pot and sear on all sides until browned.

5. Add the garlic, half of the tomatoes, chicken stock, orange juice, and lime juice to the pot.

6. Cover the pressure cooker and cook on high pressure for 20 minutes. Once cooking is complete, let pressure release naturally.

7. Carefully remove the pressure lid and shred the pork with 2 forks.

8. Divide the cauliflower rice, pulled pork, remaining tomatoes, and onion evenly between 4 containers. Divide shredded lettuce between 4 plastic bags.

STORAGE: Once cooled, store in covered containers in the refrigerator for up to 5 days. To reheat, microwave for 2 to 3 minutes. Top with the shredded lettuce and enjoy!

COOKING HACK: If you do not have a pressure cooker, you can make this recipe in a slow cooker. Cook on high for 3 to 4 hours, or on low for 6 to 8 hours. If your slow cooker does not have a sauté setting, do steps 2 through 4 on the stovetop. For crispy carnitas, arrange the cooked and shredded pork on a foil-lined baking sheet and broil for 5 to 8 minutes, until pork begins to crisp and the top starts to brown.

Per Serving (1 container): Calories: 313; Fat: 12g; Protein: 32g; Total Carbs: 22g; Fiber: 8g; Sodium: 518mg; Iron: 4g

Zoodles with Meatballs and Pesto Sauce

Serves 4 — Prep time: 15 minutes — Cook time: 35 minutes

I am always asked where I get inspiration for my recipes. The answer is: From all over! Sometimes I can't even track the inspiration; an idea just comes to me. That is exactly how I came up with this recipe. Pesto is a personal favorite of mine, thanks to our first trip to Italy years ago. I developed a Paleo pesto recipe and decided it would pair perfectly with meatballs. Vibrant and full of flavor, the pesto pulls this whole dish together.

½ cup Pesto Sauce (page 94)

3 zucchini

½ pound ground beef

1 egg yolk

2 tablespoons almond flour

¼ teaspoon dried oregano

⅛ teaspoon onion powder

⅛ teaspoon garlic powder

⅛ teaspoon sea salt

⅛ teaspoon freshly ground black pepper

1 tablespoon extra-virgin olive oil

1. Prepare the pesto sauce and set aside.
2. Preheat the oven to 425°F.
3. Using a vegetable spiralizer or julienne peeler, create thin noodles from the zucchini.
4. In a large bowl, combine the ground beef, egg yolk, almond flour, oregano, onion powder, garlic powder, salt, and pepper.
5. Form the ground beef mixture into meatballs and put them on a foil-lined baking sheet.
6. Put the baking sheet with the meatballs in the oven and bake for about 30 minutes, until cooked through.
7. While the meatballs are cooking, heat the olive oil in a large pan over medium-high heat. Add the zucchini noodles and cook for 3 to 5 minutes, stirring with tongs until they are slightly softened.

8. Add the meatballs and pesto sauce to the pan with the zucchini noodles, and use tongs to carefully mix, making sure to coat the noodles and meatballs evenly with the pesto.

9. Divide the noodles and meatballs evenly between 4 containers.

STORAGE: Once cooled, store in covered containers in the refrigerator for up to 5 days. To reheat, microwave for 2 to 3 minutes.

SIMPLE SWAP: Change up your meatball recipe easily by swapping in ½ pound of ground turkey.

Per Serving (1 container): Calories: 376; Fat: 30g; Protein: 20g; Total Carbs: 8g; Fiber: 3g; Sodium: 148mg; Iron: 4g

Korean-Style Beef and Broccoli Bowl

Serves 4 — Prep time: 40 minutes — Cook time: 10 minutes

I like to jazz up my weekly meal prep recipes by recreating takeout favorites with fresh ingredients. This version of beef and broccoli is made with ground beef and broccoli cooked in a sweet and savory sauce, served over cauliflower rice. Quick and easy, but packed with flavor. Sneak in even more veggies by adding bell peppers, carrots, or mushrooms.

Cauliflower Rice (page 95)

2 garlic cloves, chopped

2 teaspoons freshly grated ginger or ½ teaspoon ground ginger

2 teaspoons sesame oil, divided

⅓ cup coconut aminos

2 tablespoons honey

½ white onion, sliced

¼ teaspoon sea salt

1 pound ground beef

1 small head broccoli, chopped into florets

1 tablespoon sriracha

Sesame seeds, for garnish

Chopped scallions, for garnish

1. Prepare the cauliflower rice and set aside.

2. In a small bowl, combine the garlic, ginger, 1 teaspoon of sesame oil, coconut aminos, and honey in a small bowl using a whisk.

3. In a large skillet, heat the remaining sesame oil over medium heat. Add the onion and salt and cook for 5 minutes, until softened.

4. Add the ground beef to the pan, using a wooden spoon to break up the meat into small chunks. Add the broccoli florets.

5. Add the coconut aminos mixture to the meat and turn the heat to medium-high. Cook for 5 to 7 minutes, or until the meat is cooked through and the broccoli is soft.

6. Divide the cauliflower rice, beef, and broccoli evenly between 4 containers. Drizzle each with sriracha and garnish each with sesame seeds and chopped scallions.

STORAGE: Once cooled, store in covered containers in the refrigerator for up to 5 days. To reheat, microwave for 2 to 3 minutes.

Per Serving (1 container): Calories: 408; Fat: 17g; Protein: 34g; Total Carbs: 28g; Fiber: 4g; Sodium: 964mg; Iron: 4g

Meatloaf and Mashed Cauliflower

Serves 4 — Prep time: 35 minutes — Cook time: 1 hour

This is comfort food at its finest. Inspired by everyone's favorite TV dinner, this recipe has all of the flavors you know and love from growing up, but it has been elevated with fresh, whole ingredients. Add another serving of vegetables by adding roasted broccoli or carrots to this dish.

Mashed Cauliflower (page 96)

2 pounds ground beef

1 cup almond flour

2 eggs

1 (6-ounce) can tomato paste

3 garlic cloves, minced

2 tablespoons dried basil

1½ teaspoons sea salt

1 teaspoon dried oregano

1 teaspoon onion powder

Freshly ground black pepper

1. Prepare the mashed cauliflower and set aside.

2. Preheat the oven to 350°F.

3. In a large bowl, use your hands to mix together the ground beef, almond flour, eggs, tomato paste, garlic, basil, salt, oregano, onion powder, and pepper until the mixture is consistent throughout.

4. In a large glass baking pan or bread loaf pan, form the meat mixture into a rectangular loaf.

5. Bake for 1 hour, until the center is no longer pink.

6. Divide the mashed cauliflower evenly between 4 containers. Slice the meatloaf and divide between the 4 containers.

STORAGE: Once cooled, store in covered containers in the refrigerator for up to 5 days. To reheat, microwave for 3 to 4 minutes.

SIMPLE SWAP: If you are looking to pull back on red meat or just looking to switch things up, swap the ground beef for ground turkey or chicken.

Per Serving (1 container): Calories: 786; Fat: 43g; Protein: 76g; Total Carbs: 26g; Fiber: 10g; Sodium: 1728mg; Iron: 11g

Short Rib and Root Veggie Stew

Serves 4 — Prep time: 20 minutes — Cook time: 3 hours

This stew is the perfect fall dish, and this version was inspired by my favorite Asian flavors. Not only is this recipe easy to pull together, but the ingredients can be swapped based on what is available and in season. After a little prep, the stew simmers on the stove for a few hours, melding all of the flavors together with little to no hands-on effort.

3 pounds bone-in short ribs

1½ cups coconut aminos

1 cup freshly squeezed orange juice

¼ cup rice vinegar

3¼ cups water, divided

1 cup trimmed and chopped scallions

4 tablespoons fresh ginger, chopped

1 small yellow onion, roughly chopped

2 heads garlic cloves, peeled

1 cup sliced mushrooms

1 cup diced taro root

2 carrots, peeled and diced

½ butternut squash, peeled and cubed

1. Use paper towels to fully dry the short ribs and set them aside.

2. Combine the coconut aminos, orange juice, rice vinegar, ¼ cup of water, scallions, ginger, yellow onion, and garlic in a food processor or high-speed blender and puree well.

3. Add the puree and remaining 3 cups of water to a large pot or Dutch oven. Turn the heat to high and bring to a boil.

4. Add the ribs to the pot and lower the heat to a simmer. Cover and cook for 2½ hours.

5. Add the mushrooms, taro root, carrots, and butternut squash to the stew, and stir to combine. Cover and simmer for another 30 minutes.

6. Remove the rib bones from the stew and divide the stew evenly between 4 containers.

STORAGE: Once cooled, store in covered containers in the refrigerator for up to 5 days. To reheat, microwave for 3 to 4 minutes.

COOKING HACK: Want to turn this into a slow cooker meal? Reduce the water by 1 cup and add all the ingredients (meat and vegetables) to a slow cooker pot at step 3. Cook on low for 7 to 8 hours.

SMART SHOPPING: Taro is a root vegetable that can be found in the produce section of the store. If your local market does not have taro root, it can be replaced with cassava (yuca) root, parsnip, or sweet potato.

Per Serving (1 container): Calories: 1112; Fat: 64g; Protein: 60g; Total Carbs: 63g; Fiber: 5g; Sodium: 2808mg; Iron: 9g

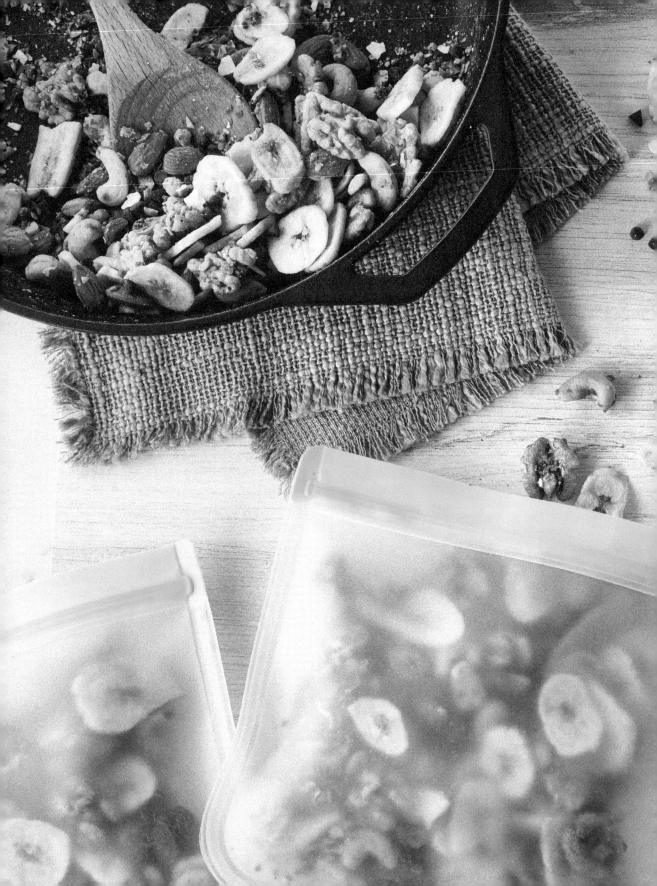

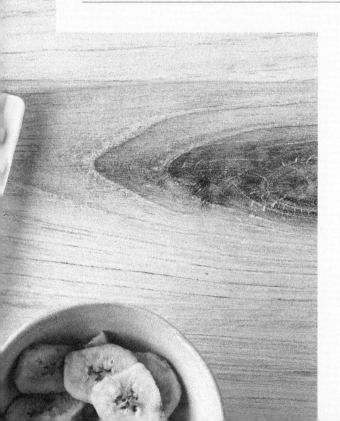

Snacks

Almond Butter Bars

Makes 16 — Prep time: 20 minutes, plus 1 hour freezing

These gluten- and grain-free Almond Butter Bars taste like dessert but can be enjoyed for breakfast or anytime as a snack. The reason I love these bars so much, besides the fact that they are made from just 5 ingredients, is the salty-sweet combo. Not to mention they are packed with protein from the almond butter. If you prefer, you can also substitute the almond butter with sunflower butter or another nut butter of your choice.

Almond Butter (page 91), divided

¼ cup, plus 2 tablespoons maple syrup

½ cup coconut flour

1 cup dark chocolate chips, melted

¼ teaspoon sea salt

1. Prepare the almond butter and set aside.

2. Line an 8-inch square baking pan with parchment paper and set aside.

3. In a mixing bowl, mix 1 cup almond butter, maple syrup, and coconut flour until well combined. Transfer the mixture to the prepared baking pan and smooth the top.

4. In a separate bowl, combine the melted chocolate chips, salt, and remaining almond butter. Transfer the chocolate mixture to the pan to create a smooth top layer.

5. Tap the pan on the counter a few times to release air pockets and even out the mixture.

6. Put the baking pan in the freezer for 1 hour, until the bars harden.

7. Once hardened, use a sharp knife to slice into 16 squares.

8. Divide bites between 8 airtight containers or plastic bags.

STORAGE: Store in covered containers in the refrigerator for up to 2 weeks, or the freezer for up to 2 months.

COOKING HACK: To melt the chocolate chips, put them in a microwave-safe bowl. Put the bowl and a mug of water in the microwave and heat in 15-second increments, until smooth and melted. Stir between intervals. The mug of water will keep the chocolate from drying out.

Per Serving (2 squares): Calories: 487; Fat: 35g; Protein: 13g; Total Carbs: 35g; Fiber: 11g; Sodium: 115mg; Iron: 5g

Chocolate Chip Cookie Dough Bites

Makes 12 — Prep time: 20 minutes

These tasty bites are the perfect snack when you want to reach for something sweet. Plus, this is a no-bake recipe, so they are super simple and quick to pull together. You can customize the flavor by adding spices like cinnamon and nutmeg and swapping the chocolate chips for nuts and raisins.

1½ cups blanched almond flour

2 tablespoons coconut flour

3 tablespoons maple syrup

2 tablespoons melted coconut oil

1½ teaspoons pure vanilla extract

½ cup dark chocolate chips

1. In a food processor, combine the almond flour, coconut flour, maple syrup, coconut oil, and vanilla extract. Pulse to combine. Add chocolate chips and fold in.

2. Line a baking sheet with parchment paper.

3. Roll a tablespoon of dough into a ball and place it on the prepared baking sheet. Repeat with remaining dough and let sit for about 5 minutes.

4. Divide bites between 6 airtight containers or plastic bags.

STORAGE: Store in covered containers for up to 7 days.

SIMPLE SWAP: Add extra protein to these Chocolate Chip Cookie Dough Bites by adding 2 tablespoons of vanilla protein powder or almond butter to the dough.

Per Serving (1 container): Calories: 330; Fat: 25g; Protein: 7g; Total Carbs: 21g; Fiber: 6g; Sodium: 12mg; Iron: 3g

Banana Coconut Trail Mix

Makes 2 cups — Prep time: 5 minutes — Cook time: 40 minutes

I used to think that trail mix was just the combination of raw nuts, seeds, and raisins, but then I realized that by toasting the nuts you are able to extract so much more flavor than I could have imagined. I love how the toasted nuts, combined with sweet coconut flakes, rich chocolate, and crunchy banana chips come together in this trail mix. Be sure to portion it out or you may eat it all in one sitting!

2 tablespoons coconut oil

1 cup raw cashews

1 cup slivered or chopped raw almonds

1 cup halved raw walnuts

½ cup unsweetened coconut flakes

1 teaspoon vanilla

2 tablespoons coconut sugar

½ tablespoon cinnamon

1½ cups unsweetened banana chips

½ cup dark chocolate chips

1. In a large skillet, heat the coconut oil over medium heat.

2. Add the cashews, almonds, walnuts, and coconut flakes to the skillet and toast uncovered for 10 minutes.

3. Add the vanilla, coconut sugar, and cinnamon to the skillet and stir to combine. Reduce the heat to low and cook for 20 minutes. Add the banana chips and cook for another 10 minutes.

4. Remove the skillet from the stove and let it cool.

5. When the skillet has cooled, add the chocolate chips and toss to mix well.

6. Divide the trail mix between 8 airtight containers or plastic bags.

STORAGE: Store for up to 2 weeks.

SIMPLE SWAP: You can easily adjust the types of nuts in this recipe as long as you keep to 3 cups of nuts. Pecans and hazelnuts work great.

Per Serving (¼ cup): Calories: 545; Fat: 44g; Protein: 11g; Total Carbs: 32g; Fiber: 10g; Sodium: 7mg; Iron: 4g

Buffalo Chicken Deviled Eggs

Makes 12 — Prep time: 20 minutes — Cook time: 15 minutes

Deviled eggs are a quick snack you can easily make Paleo friendly. This version swaps the traditional filling for buffalo chicken. Prep them in advance and store in an airtight container so you can nibble on them throughout the week.

1 pound boneless, skinless chicken breasts

½ cup chicken stock

Sea salt

Freshly ground black pepper

6 eggs

¼ cup hot sauce

½ tablespoon ghee, melted

½ teaspoon apple cider vinegar

Pinch cayenne pepper

Chopped scallions, for garnish

1. Put the chicken and chicken stock in a pressure cooker. Season with salt and pepper. Cover the pressure cooker and cook on high pressure for 8 minutes. Once cooking is complete, let the pressure release naturally.

2. Meanwhile, bring a pot of water to a boil. Put the eggs in the pot and continue to boil for 10 minutes. After removing the eggs, immediately put them in an ice bath and chill for 5 minutes.

3. Carefully remove the pressure lid and shred the chicken with 2 forks.

4. Once the eggs have cooled, peel them, cut them in half lengthwise, and scoop out the yolks and set them aside.

5. In a mixing bowl whisk together the hot sauce, ghee, apple cider vinegar, and cayenne pepper. Add the yolks to the mixture and stir to combine.

6. Toss the shredded chicken in the buffalo sauce and set aside.

7. Assemble the deviled eggs by dividing the chicken mixture between each of the 12 egg halves. Garnish each deviled egg with scallions.

8. Divide the eggs between 6 containers.

STORAGE: Once cooled, store in covered containers in the refrigerator for up to 5 days.

SIMPLE SWAP: There is an endless variety of fillings that can be used in deviled eggs. Try omitting the chicken and buffalo sauce in place of a scoop of avocado oil mayonnaise and mashed avocado.

COOKING HACK: If you do not have a pressure cooker, you can complete step 1 in a slow cooker. Cook on high for 3 to 4 hours, or low for 6 to 8 hours.

Per Serving (2 eggs): Calories: 177; Fat: 8g; Protein: 23g; Total Carbs: 2g; Fiber: 0g; Sodium: 413mg; Iron: 1g

BLT Bites

Makes 4 — Prep time: 15 minutes — Cook time: 30 minutes

These BLT bites are a play on a traditional BLT, but here the B becomes the vessel for the L and T. The combination of crunchy bacon, crisp lettuce, and bright tomatoes means you get the perfect combination in every bite. Enjoy as an afternoon snack or double the batch as a simple appetizer for your next party.

Coconut oil, for greasing

8 bacon slices, halved

2 cups chopped butter or romaine lettuce

1 tomato, diced

1. Preheat the oven to 350°F and line a baking sheet with parchment paper.

2. Turn a muffin tin upside down and grease the bottom of each cup with coconut oil.

3. Place 1 piece of bacon across the bottom of a muffin tin cup. Place a second piece of bacon across the muffin tin cup in the opposite direction. Repeat with remaining bacon until there are 8 total muffin tin cups topped with bacon.

4. Place a second muffin tin on top of the upside-down muffin tin to hold the bacon. Put both muffin tins on the prepared baking sheet.

5. Bake for 20 to 25 minutes. Remove the top muffin tin and bake for an additional 5 minutes.

6. Let cool and then top each bacon cup with chopped lettuce and tomato.

7. Divide between 4 airtight containers.

STORAGE: Store in covered containers in the refrigerator for up to 5 days.

COOKING HACK: Top these BLT bites with your favorite Paleo-friendly dressing or sauce. I like to mix a pinch of chili powder, smoked paprika, and chipotle powder with homemade mayo and a squeeze of lime juice.

Per Serving (1 container): Calories: 115; Fat: 9g; Protein: 6g; Total Carbs: 2g; Fiber: 1g; Sodium: 273mg; Iron: 1g

Grain-Free Crackers

Serves 4 — Prep time: 15 minutes — Cook time: 15 minutes

While homemade crackers may sound intimidating, these grain-free crackers are as tasty as they are easy to make. I use garlic powder to add a little extra kick, but you can swap out the garlic powder for onion powder and dill, fresh rosemary and thyme, or another seasoning of your choice.

2 cups blanched almond flour, plus more for dusting

2 eggs, lightly beaten, divided

½ teaspoon sea salt

½ teaspoon freshly ground black pepper

½ teaspoon garlic powder, optional

1 teaspoon water

1. Preheat the oven to 350°F and line 2 baking sheets with parchment paper.

2. In a food processor, combine the flour, 1 egg, salt, pepper, and garlic powder. Pulse to form a dough ball.

3. Divide the dough into 2 balls and roll out each ball to ¹⁄₁₆-inch thick on a floured surface.

4. Transfer each piece of dough to a lined baking sheet.

5. Mix together the remaining egg and the water. Lightly brush the dough with the egg wash and sprinkle with additional salt and pepper.

6. Using a sharp knife or pizza cutter, cut the dough into 1-inch squares.

7. Bake for 10 to 12 minutes, until golden brown.

8. Let cool and divide between 4 airtight containers or plastic bags.

STORAGE: Once cooled, store in covered containers in the refrigerator for up to 5 days.

COOKING HACK: Keep the counter clean and instead roll out the dough between two pieces of parchment paper. If you do not have a food processor, you can combine ingredients in a mixing bowl by hand.

Per Serving (1 container): Calories: 356; Fat: 31g; Protein: 15g; Total Carbs: 11g; Fiber: 6g; Sodium: 328mg; Iron: 2g

Beef Jerky

Serves 4 — Prep time: 20 minutes, plus 2 hours for freezing and overnight marinating — Cook time: 4 hours

Many beef jerky recipes call for the use of a dehydrator, but there is no fancy equipment needed for this recipe. In fact, this recipe calls for just a handful of simple ingredients and an oven to create savory homemade beef jerky. Salty, sweet, and smoky, this jerky is packed with flavor.

1 pound flank steak

2 garlic cloves, minced

⅓ cup coconut aminos

2 tablespoons maple syrup

½ teaspoon freshly ground black pepper

½ teaspoon salt

½ teaspoon onion powder

½ teaspoon garlic powder

½ teaspoon smoked paprika

½ teaspoon chipotle powder

1. Freeze the flank steak for about 2 hours, until firm.

2. Trim any visible fat from the steak and slice into thin strips, about ⅛ inch thick.

3. In a mixing bowl, whisk together the remaining ingredients. Place the sliced steak and marinade into a shallow dish or plastic bag. Put in the refrigerator and let marinate overnight.

4. Preheat the oven to 170°F and line 2 baking sheets with parchment paper. Put a wire cooling rack on top of each baking sheet.

5. Meanwhile, remove the meat from the refrigerator and pat it dry with paper towels. Arrange the meat evenly on the rack so that they are not touching. Cook for 4 hours, turning halfway through, until dry.

6. Let cool and divide between 4 airtight containers or plastic bags.

STORAGE: Store in a cool place or refrigerator for up to 7 days.

COOKING HACK: To keep the air circulating, cook with the oven door open a crack. Do not use the convection setting on your oven, as the fan speed will be too high.

Per Serving (1 container): Calories: 256; Fat: 5g; Protein: 34g; Total Carbs: 17g; Fiber: 0g; Sodium: 638mg; Iron: 3g

Fruit Leather

Makes 10 — Prep time: 15 minutes — Cook time: 3 to 4 hours

Growing up, gummy snacks were my absolute favorite treat, and I loved finding a Fruit by the Foot inside of my lunch box. This homemade version is made from just three simple ingredients—strawberries as the base, honey for a hint of sweetness, and lemon juice to balance the flavor. Try variations of this recipe by swapping out the strawberries for another berry of your choice or a mix of berries. Strawberry is my favorite, but my husband loves half-strawberry, half-raspberry. Blueberries, blackberries, and cranberries also work well.

4 cups strawberries, hulled

2 tablespoons honey

1 teaspoon freshly squeezed lemon juice

1. Preheat the oven to 170°F and line 2 baking sheets with parchment paper.
2. In a high-speed blender, blend the strawberries, honey, and lemon juice until smooth.
3. Pour the strawberry puree onto the center of the lined baking sheets, and use a spatula to spread evenly without leaving any translucent spots.
4. Cook for 3 to 4 hours, until the center is no longer sticky. Check every 30 minutes to ensure the fruit leather is dehydrated but not burned.
5. Let cool and then remove the parchment paper from the baking sheet. Cut the fruit leather into strips.
6. Divide between 10 airtight containers or plastic bags.

STORAGE: Store in a cool place or refrigerator for up to 7 days.

COOKING HACK: If you have a nonstick baking mat, swap the parchment paper for the baking mat.

Per Serving (1 container): Calories: 41; Fat: 0g; Protein: 1g; Total Carbs: 10g; Fiber: 2g; Sodium: 1mg; Iron: 0g

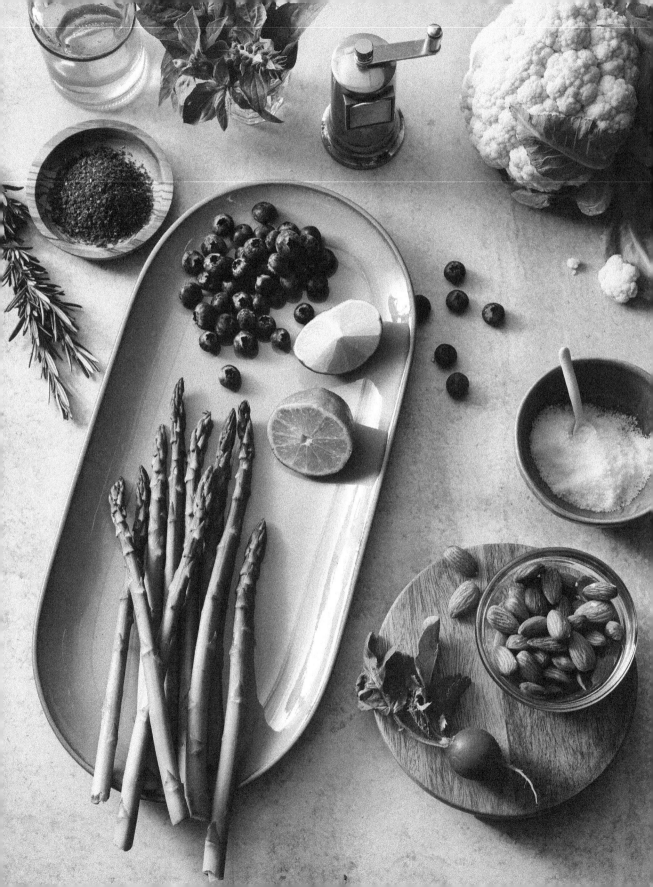

Measurement Conversions

VOLUME EQUIVALENTS (LIQUID)

US Standard	US Standard (ounces)	Metric (approximate)
2 tablespoons	1 fl. oz.	30 mL
¼ cup	2 fl. oz.	60 mL
½ cup	4 fl. oz.	120 mL
1 cup	8 fl. oz.	240 mL
1½ cups	12 fl. oz.	355 mL
2 cups or 1 pint	16 fl. oz.	475 mL
4 cups or 1 quart	32 fl. oz.	1 L
1 gallon	128 fl. oz.	4 L

OVEN TEMPERATURES

Fahrenheit (F)	Celsius (C) (approximate)
250°F	120°C
300°F	150°C
325°F	165°C
350°F	180°C
375°F	190°C
400°F	200°C
425°F	220°C
450°F	230°C

VOLUME EQUIVALENTS (DRY)

US Standard	Metric (approximate)
⅛ teaspoon	0.5 mL
¼ teaspoon	1 mL
½ teaspoon	2 mL
¾ teaspoon	4 mL
1 teaspoon	5 mL
1 tablespoon	15 mL
¼ cup	59 mL
⅓ cup	79 mL
½ cup	118 mL
⅔ cup	156 mL
¾ cup	177 mL
1 cup	235 mL
2 cups or 1 pint	475 mL
3 cups	700 mL
4 cups or 1 quart	1 L

WEIGHT EQUIVALENTS

US Standard	Metric (approximate)
½ ounce	15 g
1 ounce	30 g
2 ounces	60 g
4 ounces	115 g
8 ounces	225 g
12 ounces	340 g
16 ounces or 1 pound	455 g

Index

Acknowledgments

First and foremost, thank you to Julien, my best friend, my faithful taste tester, my cameraman, and my husband. Thank you for supporting me through late nights of copywriting and long days of recipe testing.

To my friends and family: Thank you for your words of encouragement and cheering for me throughout this journey. I am so thankful to have each and every one of you in my corner.

To Rachelle and my second family at Callisto Media: Thank you for all your time and patience throughout this entire process and for your constant encouragement. I am so grateful to have had the experience of writing this book together.

Last, but not least, to you, my amazing readers. Thank you for following my journey over the past 8 years and for bringing me into your home to help you.

About the Author

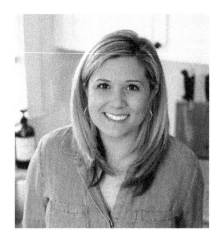

Kenzie Swanhart is a home cook turned food blogger and cookbook author, providing her readers inspiration both in and out of the kitchen. With more than 300,000 copies of her best-selling cookbooks in print, Kenzie never wavers in her mission: creating and sharing easy yet flavorful recipes made with real ingredients with her readers.

As the head of culinary innovation and marketing for Ninja, Kenzie and her team provide a unique, food-first point of view for the development of new products and recipes to make consumers' lives easier so they can be proud of what they cook. You'll also see her serving as the face of Ninja on QVC, where she shares tips, tricks, and recipes for the company's full line of products.

Kenzie lives in the Boston area with her husband, Julien, and their dog, Charlie.

CPSIA information can be obtained
at www.ICGtesting.com
Printed in the USA
JSHW040002290620
6379JS00002B/39